Case No. _____

Veterinary Patient Organizer / SOAP Notebook / History & Physical Exam Templates

By. Lance Wheeler

Case No. _____

By. Lance Wheeler

Property of: _____

Phone No.: _____

Date: _____

Table of Contents

Page	Case No.	Patient	Admit Date	Problem
4				
8				
12				
16				
20				
24				
28				
32				
36				
40				
44				
48				
52				
56				
60				
64				
68				
72				
76				
80				
84				
88				
92				
96				
100				
104				
108				
112				
116				
120				
124				
128				
132				
136				
140				
144				
148				
152				
156				
160				
164				
168				
172				

"It's not that I'm so smart, but I stay with the questions much longer."
- Albert Einstein

Case No._____

Patient	Age	Sex		Breed		Weight
		nM	sF			
	DOB:	iM	iF	Color:		kg

Owner	Primary Veterinarian	Admit Date/ Time
Name: Phone:	Name: Phone:	Date: Time: AM / PM

• **Presenting complaint**:_____
_____
_____
_____
_____
_____

• **Medical Hx**:_____
_____
_____
_____
_____

• **When/ where obtained**: Date:_____; □Breeder, □Shelter, Other:_____

Drug/ Supplement	Amount	Dose (mg/kg)	Route	Frequency	Date Started

• **Vaccine status – Dog**: □Rab □Parv □Dist □Aden; □Para □Lep □Bord □Influ □Lyme
• **Vaccine status – Cat**: □Rab □Herp □Cali □Pan □FeLV [kittens]; □FIV □Chlam □Bord
• **Heartworm / Flea & Tick / Intestinal Parasites**:
  ◦ *Last Heartworm Test*: Date:_____, □IDK; Test Results: □Pos, □Neg, □IDK
  ◦ *Monthly heartworm preventative*: □no □yes, Product:_____
  ◦ *Monthly flea & tick preventative*: □no □yes, Product:_____
  ◦ *Monthly dewormer*:   □no □yes, Product:_____
• **Surgical Hx**: □Spay/Neuter; Date:_____; Other:_____
• **Environment**: □Indoor, □Outdoor, Time spent outdoors/ Other:_____
• **Housemates**: Dogs:_____ Cats:_____ Other:_____
• **Diet**: □Wet, □Dry; Brand/ Amt.:_____

Appetite	□Normal, □↑, □↓
Weight	□Normal, □↑, □↓; Past Wt.:_____ kg; Date:_____; Δ:_____
Thirst	□Normal, □↑, □↓
Urination	□Normal, □↑, □↓, □Blood, □Strain
Defecation	□Normal, □↑, □↓, □Blood, □Strain, □Diarrhea, □Mucus
Discharge	□No, □Yes; Onset/ Describe:
Cough/ Sneeze	□No, □Yes; Onset/ Describe:
Vomit	□No, □Yes; Onset/ Describe:
Respiration	□Normal, □↑ Rate, □↑ Effort
Energy level	□Normal, □Lethargic, □Exercise intolerance

• **Travel Hx**: □None, Other:_____
• **Exposure to**: □Standing water, □Wildlife, □Board/daycare, □Dog park, □Groomer, □Pet store
• **Adverse reactions to food/ meds**: □None, Other:_____
• **Can give oral meds**: □no □yes; Helpful Tricks:_____

Physical Exam – General:

- **Body Weight**:_____kg   **Body Condition Score**:___/9

- **Temperature**:_____°F [*Dog-RI*: 100.9–102.4; *Cat-RI*: 98.1–102.1]

- **Heart**:
  - *Rate*:_____beats/min [*Dog-RI*: 60–180; *Cat-RI*: 140–240 (in hospital)]
  - *Rhythm*: ☐Regular, ☐Irregular
  - *Sounds*: ☐None, ☐Split sound[S1 or S2], ☐Gallop[S3 or S4], ☐Murmur, ☐Muffled
    - *Grade*: ☐1–2[soft, only at PMI], ☐3–4[moderate, mild radiate], ☐5–6[loud, strong radiate, thrill]
    - *Timing*: ☐Systolic, ☐Diastolic, ☐Continuous
    - *PMI*:

	PMI	Over	Anatomic Boundaries
☐	Lt. apex	Mitral valve	5th to 6th ICS at level of CCJ
☐	Lt. base	Ao + Pul outflow	2nd to 4th ICS above the CCJ
☐	Rt. midheart	Tricuspid valve	3rd to 5th ICS near the CCJ
☐	Rt. sternal border	Right ventricle	5th to 7th ICS immediately dorsal to the sternum
☐	Sternal (cat)	Sternum	In cats, determination of PMI offers very little clinical significance.

  - • *Vertebral Heart Size*: Dog = 8.7–10.7; Cat = 6.9–8.1 (from cranial edge of T4)
  - • *Innocent Murmur*: Grade 1-2, systolic, left base location, disappear by ~4 months of age, absent clinical signs

- **Pulses**:
  - *Pulse rate*:_____pulses/min
  - *Character*: ☐Sync, ☐Async; ☐Normokinetic, ☐Hyper-, ☐Hypo-, ☐Variable

- **Lungs**:
  - *Respiratory rate*:_____breaths/min [*RI*: 16–30]
  - *Depth/Effort*: ☐Norm, ☐Pant, ☐Deep, ☐Shallow, ☐↑ Insp. effort, ☐↑ Exp. effort
  - *Sounds/Localization*:
    - ☐Norm BV, ☐Quiet BV, ☐Loud BV, ☐Crack, ☐Wheez, ☐Frict, ☐Muffled
    - ☐All lung fields, ☐Rt cran, ☐Rt mid, ☐Rt caud, ☐Lt cran, ☐Lt mid, ☐Lt caud
  - *Tracheal Auscultation/ Palpation*: ☐Normal, Other:_____

- **Pain Score**:_____ / 5   Localization:_____

- **Mentation**:

☐BAR ☐QAR ☐Dull (conscious; responds to sensory stimuli)	☐Confused/ Disoriented (conscious; inappropriate response to environment [ex., vocalization, head pressing])	☐Drowsy/ Obtunded (↓ interaction with environment; slow response to verbal stimuli)	☐Stuporous (unresponsive unless aroused by noxious stimuli)	☐Coma (complete unresponsiveness to any stimuli)

- **Skin Elasticity**: ☐Normal skin turgor, ☐↓ Skin turgor, ☐Skin tent, ☐Gelatinous

- **Mucus Membranes**:
  - *CRT*:_____ [*RI*: 1–2; <1 = compensated shock, sepsis, heat stroke; <2 = acute decompensated shock; >2 = late decompensated shock, decreased cardiac output, hypothermia]
  - *Color*:_____ [*RI*: pink; red = compensated shock, sepsis, heat stroke; pale/white = anemia, shock; blue = cyanosis; yellow = hepatic disease, extravascular hemolysis; brown = met-Hb]
  - *Texture*:_____ [*RI*: moist = hydrated; tacky-to-dry = 5–12% dehydrated]

Physical Exam – Systems Checklist:

- **Head:** _____ ☐NAF
  - ○ Ears: ☐Ceruminous debris (mild / mod / sev) (AS / AD / AU), _____ ☐NAF
  - ○ Eyes: _____ ☐NAF
    - ▪ Retinal: _____ ☐NAF

→ Ⓛ	Ⓡ	Ⓛ	Ⓡ ←
☐ ⊙ Normal Direct	☐ ⊙ Normal Indirect	☐ ⊙ Normal Indirect	☐ ⊙ Normal Direct
☐ ● Abnormal Direct	☐ ● Abnormal Indirect	☐ ● Abnormal Indirect	☐ ● Abnormal Direct

  - ○ Nose: _____ ☐NAF
  - ○ Oral cavity: ☐Tarter/Gingivitis (mild / mod / sev), _____ ☐NAF
  - ○ Mandibular lnn.: ☐Enlarged Lt., ☐Enlarged Rt., _____ ☐NAF

- **Neck:** _____ ☐NAF
  - ○ Superficial cervical lnn.: ☐Enlarged Lt., ☐Enlarged Rt., _____ ☐NAF
  - ○ Thyroid: _____ ☐NAF

- **Thoracic limb:** _____ ☐NAF
  - ○ Foot pads: _____ ☐NAF
  - ○ Knuckling: _____ ☐NAF
  - ○ Axillary lnn. [normally absent]: _____ ☐NAF

- **Thorax:** _____ ☐NAF

- **Abdomen:** _____ ☐NAF
  - ○ Mammary chain: _____ ☐NAF
  - ○ Penis/ Testicles/ Vulva: _____ ☐NAF
  - ○ Superficial inguinal lnn. [normally absent]: _____ ☐NAF

- **Pelvic limb:** _____ ☐NAF
  - ○ Foot pads: _____ ☐NAF
  - ○ Knuckling: _____ ☐NAF
  - ○ Popliteal lnn.: ☐Enlarged Lt., ☐Enlarged Rt., _____ ☐NAF

- **Skin:** _____ ☐NAF
- **Tail:** _____ ☐NAF
- **Rectal ☞ ⊙:** _____ ☐NAF

Problems List:

- **Problem #1**:

- **Problem #2**:

- **Problem #3**:

- **Problem #4**:

- **Problem #5**:

- **Problem #6**:

Diagnostic Plan	Treatment Plan

Case No._____

Patient	Age	Sex		Breed	Weight
		nM	sF		
	DOB:	iM	iF	Color:	kg

Owner		Primary Veterinarian	Admit Date/ Time
Name: Phone:		Name: Phone:	Date: Time: AM / PM

• **Presenting complaint**:_____
_____
_____
_____
_____
_____

• **Medical Hx**:_____
_____
_____
_____
_____

• **When/ where obtained**: Date:_____; ☐Breeder, ☐Shelter, Other:_____

Drug/ Supplement	Amount	Dose (mg/kg)	Route	Frequency	Date Started

• **Vaccine status – Dog**: ☐Rab ☐Parv ☐Dist ☐Aden; ☐Para ☐Lep ☐Bord ☐Influ ☐Lyme
• **Vaccine status – Cat**: ☐Rab ☐Herp ☐Cali ☐Pan ☐FeLV [kittens]; ☐FIV ☐Chlam ☐Bord
• **Heartworm / Flea & Tick / Intestinal Parasites**:
  ◦ *Last Heartworm Test*: Date:_____, ☐IDK; Test Results: ☐Pos, ☐Neg, ☐IDK
  ◦ *Monthly heartworm preventative*: ☐no ☐yes, Product:_____
  ◦ *Monthly flea & tick preventative*: ☐no ☐yes, Product:_____
  ◦ *Monthly dewormer*: ☐no ☐yes, Product:_____
• **Surgical Hx**: ☐Spay/Neuter; Date:_____; Other:_____
• **Environment**: ☐Indoor, ☐Outdoor, Time spent outdoors/ Other:_____
• **Housemates**: Dogs:_____ Cats:_____ Other:_____
• **Diet**: ☐Wet, ☐Dry; Brand/ Amt.:_____

Appetite	☐Normal, ☐↑, ☐↓
Weight	☐Normal, ☐↑, ☐↓; Past Wt.:_____kg; Date:_____; Δ:_____
Thirst	☐Normal, ☐↑, ☐↓
Urination	☐Normal, ☐↑, ☐↓, ☐Blood, ☐Strain
Defecation	☐Normal, ☐↑, ☐↓, ☐Blood, ☐Strain, ☐Diarrhea, ☐Mucus
Discharge	☐No, ☐Yes; Onset/ Describe:
Cough/ Sneeze	☐No, ☐Yes; Onset/ Describe:
Vomit	☐No, ☐Yes; Onset/ Describe:
Respiration	☐Normal, ☐↑ Rate, ☐↑ Effort
Energy level	☐Normal, ☐Lethargic, ☐Exercise intolerance

• **Travel Hx**: ☐None, Other:_____
• **Exposure to**: ☐Standing water, ☐Wildlife, ☐Board/daycare, ☐Dog park, ☐Groomer, ☐Pet store
• **Adverse reactions to food/ meds**: ☐None, Other:_____
• **Can give oral meds**: ☐no ☐yes; Helpful Tricks:_____

Physical Exam – General:

- **Body Weight**:_____ kg **Body Condition Score**:___ /9

- **Temperature**:_____ °F [*Dog-RI*: 100.9–102.4; *Cat-RI*: 98.1–102.1]

- **Heart**:
  - *Rate*:_____ beats/min [Dog-RI: 60–180; Cat-RI: 140–240 (in hospital)]
  - *Rhythm*: ☐Regular, ☐Irregular
  - *Sounds*: ☐None, ☐Split sound[S1 or S2], ☐Gallop[S3 or S4], ☐Murmur, ☐Muffled
    - *Grade*: ☐1–2[soft, only at PMI], ☐3–4[moderate, mild radiate], ☐5–6[loud, strong radiate, thrill]
    - *Timing*: ☐Systolic, ☐Diastolic, ☐Continuous
    - *PMI*:

	PMI	Over	Anatomic Boundaries
☐	Lt. apex	Mitral valve	5th to 6th ICS at level of CCJ
☐	Lt. base	Ao + Pul outflow	2nd to 4th ICS above the CCJ
☐	Rt. midheart	Tricuspid valve	3rd to 5th ICS near the CCJ
☐	Rt. sternal border	Right ventricle	5th to 7th ICS immediately dorsal to the sternum
☐	Sternal (cat)	Sternum	In cats, determination of PMI offers very little clinical significance.

  - *Vertebral Heart Size*: Dog = 8.7–10.7; Cat = 6.9–8.1 (from cranial edge of T4)
  - *Innocent Murmur*: Grade 1-2, systolic, left base location, disappear by ~4 months of age, absent clinical signs

- **Pulses**:
  - *Pulse rate*:_____ pulses/min
  - *Character*: ☐Sync, ☐Async; ☐Normokinetic, ☐Hyper-, ☐Hypo-, ☐Variable

- **Lungs**:
  - *Respiratory rate*:_____ breaths/min [*RI*: 16–30]
  - *Depth/Effort*: ☐Norm, ☐Pant, ☐Deep, ☐Shallow, ☐↑ Insp. effort, ☐↑ Exp. effort
  - *Sounds/Localization*:
    - ☐Norm BV, ☐Quiet BV, ☐Loud BV, ☐Crack, ☐Wheez, ☐Frict, ☐Muffled
    - ☐All lung fields, ☐Rt cran, ☐Rt mid, ☐Rt caud, ☐Lt cran, ☐Lt mid, ☐Lt caud
  - *Tracheal Auscultation/ Palpation*: ☐Normal, Other:_____

- **Pain Score**:_____ / 5   Localization:_____

- **Mentation**:

☐BAR ☐QAR ☐Dull (conscious; responds to sensory stimuli)	☐Confused/ Disoriented (conscious; inappropriate response to environment [ex., vocalization, head pressing])	☐Drowsy/ Obtunded (↓ interaction with environment; slow response to verbal stimuli)	☐Stuporous (unresponsive unless aroused by noxious stimuli)	☐Coma (complete unresponsiveness to any stimuli)

- **Skin Elasticity**: ☐Normal skin turgor, ☐↓ Skin turgor, ☐Skin tent, ☐Gelatinous

- **Mucus Membranes**:
  - *CRT*:_____ [*RI*: 1–2; <1 = compensated shock, sepsis, heat stroke; <2 = acute decompensated shock; >2 = late decompensated shock, decreased cardiac output, hypothermia]
  - *Color*:_____ [*RI*: pink; red = compensated shock, sepsis, heat stroke; pale/white = anemia, shock; blue = cyanosis; yellow = hepatic disease, extravascular hemolysis; brown = met-Hb]
  - *Texture*:_____ [*RI*: moist = hydrated; tacky-to-dry = 5–12% dehydrated]

Physical Exam – Systems Checklist:

- Head:_____ ☐NAF
  - Ears: ☐Ceruminous debris (mild / mod / sev) (AS / AD / AU), _____ ☐NAF
  - Eyes:_____ ☐NAF
    - Retinal:_____ ☐NAF

→ Ⓛ		Ⓡ		Ⓛ		Ⓡ ←	
☐ ⊙ Normal Direct	☐ ⊙ Normal Indirect	☐ ⊙ Normal Indirect	☐ ⊙ Normal Direct
☐ ⊙ Abnormal Direct	☐ ⊙ Abnormal Indirect	☐ ⊙ Abnormal Indirect	☐ ⊙ Abnormal Direct

  - Nose:_____ ☐NAF
  - Oral cavity: ☐Tarter/Gingivitis (mild / mod / sev), _____ ☐NAF
  - Mandibular lnn.: ☐Enlarged Lt., ☐Enlarged Rt., _____ ☐NAF

- Neck:_____ ☐NAF
  - Superficial cervical lnn.: ☐Enlarged Lt., ☐Enlarged Rt., _____ ☐NAF
  - Thyroid:_____ ☐NAF

- Thoracic limb:_____ ☐NAF
  - Foot pads:_____ ☐NAF
  - Knuckling:_____ ☐NAF
  - Axillary lnn. [normally absent]:_____ ☐NAF

- Thorax:_____ ☐NAF

- Abdomen:_____ ☐NAF
  - Mammary chain:_____ ☐NAF
  - Penis/ Testicles/ Vulva:_____ ☐NAF
  - Superficial inguinal lnn. [normally absent]:_____ ☐NAF

- Pelvic limb:_____ ☐NAF
  - Foot pads:_____ ☐NAF
  - Knuckling:_____ ☐NAF
  - Popliteal lnn.: ☐Enlarged Lt., ☐Enlarged Rt., _____ ☐NAF

- Skin:_____ ☐NAF
- Tail:_____ ☐NAF
- Rectal☞☉:_____ ☐NAF

Problems List:

- **Problem #1:**

- **Problem #2:**

- **Problem #3:**

- **Problem #4:**

- **Problem #5:**

- **Problem #6:**

Diagnostic Plan	Treatment Plan

Case No._____

Patient	Age	Sex		Breed		Weight
		nM	sF			
	DOB:	iM	iF	Color:		kg

Owner	Primary Veterinarian	Admit Date/ Time
Name: Phone:	Name: Phone:	Date: Time: AM / PM

• **Presenting complaint**:_____
_____
_____
_____
_____
_____

• **Medical Hx**:_____
_____
_____
_____
_____

• **When/ where obtained**: Date:_____; □Breeder, □Shelter, Other:_____

Drug/ Supplement	Amount	Dose (mg/kg)	Route	Frequency	Date Started

• **Vaccine status – Dog**: □Rab □Parv □Dist □Aden; □Para □Lep □Bord □Influ □Lyme
• **Vaccine status – Cat**: □Rab □Herp □Cali □Pan □FeLV [kittens]; □FIV □Chlam □Bord
• **Heartworm / Flea & Tick / Intestinal Parasites**:
  ◦ *Last Heartworm Test*: Date:_____, □IDK; Test Results: □Pos, □Neg, □IDK
  ◦ *Monthly heartworm preventative*: □no □yes, Product:_____
  ◦ *Monthly flea & tick preventative*: □no □yes, Product:_____
  ◦ *Monthly dewormer*:   □no □yes, Product:_____
• **Surgical Hx**: □Spay/Neuter; Date:_____; Other:_____
• **Environment**: □Indoor, □Outdoor, Time spent outdoors/ Other:_____
• **Housemates**: Dogs:_____ Cats:_____ Other:_____
• **Diet**: □Wet, □Dry; Brand/ Amt.:_____

Appetite	□Normal, □↑, □↓
Weight	□Normal, □↑, □↓; Past Wt.:_____ kg; Date:_____; Δ:_____
Thirst	□Normal, □↑, □↓
Urination	□Normal, □↑, □↓, □Blood, □Strain
Defecation	□Normal, □↑, □↓, □Blood, □Strain, □Diarrhea, □Mucus
Discharge	□No, □Yes; Onset/ Describe:
Cough/ Sneeze	□No, □Yes; Onset/ Describe:
Vomit	□No, □Yes; Onset/ Describe:
Respiration	□Normal, □↑ Rate, □↑ Effort
Energy level	□Normal, □Lethargic, □Exercise intolerance

• **Travel Hx**: □None, Other:_____
• **Exposure to**: □Standing water, □Wildlife, □Board/daycare, □Dog park, □Groomer, □Pet store
• **Adverse reactions to food/ meds**: □None, Other:_____
• **Can give oral meds**: □no □yes; Helpful Tricks:_____

Physical Exam – General:

- **Body Weight**:_____kg   **Body Condition Score**:___/9

- **Temperature**:_____°F [*Dog-RI*: 100.9–102.4; *Cat-RI*: 98.1–102.1]

- **Heart**:
  - *Rate*:_____beats/min [Dog-RI: 60–180; Cat-RI: 140–240 (in hospital)]
  - *Rhythm*: ☐Regular, ☐Irregular
  - *Sounds*: ☐None, ☐Split sound[S1 or S2], ☐Gallop[S3 or S4], ☐Murmur, ☐Muffled
    - *Grade*: ☐1–2[soft, only at PMI],   ☐3–4[moderate, mild radiate],   ☐5–6[loud, strong radiate, thrill]
    - *Timing*: ☐Systolic, ☐Diastolic, ☐Continuous
    - *PMI*:

	PMI	Over	Anatomic Boundaries
☐	Lt. apex	Mitral valve	5th to 6th ICS at level of CCJ
☐	Lt. base	Ao + Pul outflow	2nd to 4th ICS above the CCJ
☐	Rt. midheart	Tricuspid valve	3rd to 5th ICS near the CCJ
☐	Rt. sternal border	Right ventricle	5th to 7th ICS immediately dorsal to the sternum
☐	Sternal (cat)	Sternum	In cats, determination of PMI offers very little clinical significance.

  - • *Vertebral Heart Size*: Dog = 8.7–10.7; Cat = 6.9–8.1 (from cranial edge of T4)
  - • *Innocent Murmur*: Grade 1-2, systolic, left base location, disappear by ~4 months of age, absent clinical signs

- **Pulses**:
  - *Pulse rate*:_____pulses/min
  - *Character*:   ☐Sync, ☐Async;   ☐Normokinetic, ☐Hyper-, ☐Hypo-, ☐Variable

- **Lungs**:
  - *Respiratory rate*:_____breaths/min [*RI*: 16–30]
  - *Depth/Effort*: ☐Norm, ☐Pant, ☐Deep, ☐Shallow, ☐↑ Insp. effort, ☐↑ Exp. effort
  - *Sounds/Localization*:
    - ☐Norm BV, ☐Quiet BV, ☐Loud BV, ☐Crack, ☐Wheez, ☐Frict, ☐Muffled
    - ☐All lung fields, ☐Rt cran, ☐Rt mid, ☐Rt caud, ☐Lt cran, ☐Lt mid, ☐Lt caud
  - *Tracheal Auscultation/ Palpation*: ☐Normal, Other:_____

- **Pain Score**:_____ / 5   Localization:_____

- **Mentation**: ☐BAR   ☐Confused/   ☐Drowsy/   ☐Stuporous   ☐Coma
               ☐QAR   Disoriented   Obtunded   (unresponsive unless   (complete
               ☐Dull   (conscious; inappropriate (↓ interaction with   aroused by noxious   unresponsiveness
               (conscious; responds   response to environment   environment; slow   stimuli)   to any stimuli)
               to sensory stimuli)   [ex., vocalization, head   response to verbal
                                     pressing])   stimuli)

- **Skin Elasticity**: ☐Normal skin turgor, ☐↓ Skin turgor, ☐Skin tent, ☐Gelatinous

- **Mucus Membranes**:
  - *CRT*:_____ [*RI*: 1–2; <1 = compensated shock, sepsis, heat stroke; <2 = acute decompensated shock;
                      >2 = late decompensated shock, decreased cardiac output, hypothermia]
  - *Color*:_____ [*RI*: pink; red = compensated shock, sepsis, heat stroke; pale/white = anemia, shock;
                        blue = cyanosis; yellow = hepatic disease, extravascular hemolysis; brown = met-Hb]
  - *Texture*:_____ [*RI*: moist = hydrated; tacky-to-dry = 5–12% dehydrated]

Physical Exam – Systems Checklist:

- Head:_____ ☐NAF
  - ◦ Ears: ☐Ceruminous debris (mild / mod / sev) (AS / AD / AU), _____ ☐NAF
  - ◦ Eyes:_____ ☐NAF
    - ▪ Retinal:_____ ☐NAF

→ Ⓛ		Ⓡ		Ⓛ		Ⓡ ←	
☐	⊙ Normal Direct	☐	⊙ Normal Indirect	☐	⊙ Normal Indirect	☐	⊙ Normal Direct
☐	◉ Abnormal Direct	☐	◉ Abnormal Indirect	☐	◉ Abnormal Indirect	☐	◉ Abnormal Direct

  - ◦ Nose:_____ ☐NAF
  - ◦ Oral cavity: ☐Tarter/Gingivitis (mild / mod / sev), _____ ☐NAF
  - ◦ Mandibular lnn.: ☐Enlarged Lt., ☐Enlarged Rt., _____ ☐NAF

- Neck:_____ ☐NAF
  - ◦ Superficial cervical lnn.: ☐Enlarged Lt., ☐Enlarged Rt., _____ ☐NAF
  - ◦ Thyroid:_____ ☐NAF

- Thoracic limb:_____ ☐NAF
  - ◦ Foot pads:_____ ☐NAF
  - ◦ Knuckling:_____ ☐NAF
  - ◦ Axillary lnn. [normally absent]:_____ ☐NAF

- Thorax:_____ ☐NAF

- Abdomen:_____ ☐NAF
  - ◦ Mammary chain:_____ ☐NAF
  - ◦ Penis/ Testicles/ Vulva:_____ ☐NAF
  - ◦ Superficial inguinal lnn. [normally absent]:_____ ☐NAF

- Pelvic limb:_____ ☐NAF
  - ◦ Foot pads:_____ ☐NAF
  - ◦ Knuckling:_____ ☐NAF
  - ◦ Popliteal lnn.: ☐Enlarged Lt., ☐Enlarged Rt., _____ ☐NAF

- Skin:_____ ☐NAF
- Tail:_____ ☐NAF
- Rectal☞⊙:_____ ☐NAF

14

Problems List:

- **Problem #1**:

- **Problem #2**:

- **Problem #3**:

- **Problem #4**:

- **Problem #5**:

- **Problem #6**:

Diagnostic Plan	Treatment Plan

Patient	Age	Sex		Breed		Weight
		nM	sF			
	DOB:	iM	iF	Color:		kg

Owner	Primary Veterinarian	Admit Date/ Time
Name: Phone:	Name: Phone:	Date: Time: AM / PM

• **Presenting complaint**:_____

_____

_____

_____

_____

• **Medical Hx**:_____

_____

_____

_____

• **When/ where obtained**: Date:_____; ☐Breeder, ☐Shelter, Other:_____

Drug/ Supplement	Amount	Dose (mg/kg)	Route	Frequency	Date Started

• **Vaccine status – Dog**: ☐Rab ☐Parv ☐Dist ☐Aden; ☐Para ☐Lep ☐Bord ☐Influ ☐Lyme
• **Vaccine status – Cat**: ☐Rab ☐Herp ☐Cali ☐Pan ☐FeLV [kittens]; ☐FIV ☐Chlam ☐Bord
• **Heartworm / Flea & Tick / Intestinal Parasites**:
  ◦ *Last Heartworm Test*: Date:_____, ☐IDK; Test Results: ☐Pos, ☐Neg, ☐IDK
  ◦ *Monthly heartworm preventative*: ☐no ☐yes, Product:_____
  ◦ *Monthly flea & tick preventative*: ☐no ☐yes, Product:_____
  ◦ *Monthly dewormer*:   ☐no ☐yes, Product:_____
• **Surgical Hx**: ☐Spay/Neuter; Date:_____; Other:_____
• **Environment**: ☐Indoor, ☐Outdoor, Time spent outdoors/ Other:_____
• **Housemates**: Dogs:_____ Cats:_____ Other:_____
• **Diet**: ☐Wet, ☐Dry; Brand/ Amt.:_____

Appetite	☐Normal, ☐↑, ☐↓
Weight	☐Normal, ☐↑, ☐↓; Past Wt.:_____ kg; Date:_____; Δ:_____
Thirst	☐Normal, ☐↑, ☐↓
Urination	☐Normal, ☐↑, ☐↓, ☐Blood, ☐Strain
Defecation	☐Normal, ☐↑, ☐↓, ☐Blood, ☐Strain, ☐Diarrhea, ☐Mucus
Discharge	☐No, ☐Yes; Onset/ Describe:
Cough/ Sneeze	☐No, ☐Yes; Onset/ Describe:
Vomit	☐No, ☐Yes; Onset/ Describe:
Respiration	☐Normal, ☐↑ Rate, ☐↑ Effort
Energy level	☐Normal, ☐Lethargic, ☐Exercise intolerance

• **Travel Hx**: ☐None, Other:_____
• **Exposure to**: ☐Standing water, ☐Wildlife, ☐Board/daycare, ☐Dog park, ☐Groomer, ☐Pet store
• **Adverse reactions to food/ meds**: ☐None, Other:_____
• **Can give oral meds**: ☐no ☐yes; Helpful Tricks:_____

Physical Exam – General:

- **Body Weight:**_____kg   **Body Condition Score:**___/9

- **Temperature:**_____°F [*Dog-RI*: 100.9–102.4; *Cat-RI*: 98.1–102.1]

- **Heart:**
  - *Rate:*_____beats/min [Dog-RI: 60–180; Cat-RI: 140–240 (in hospital)]
  - *Rhythm:* □Regular, □Irregular
  - *Sounds:* □None, □Split sound[S1 or S2], □Gallop[S3 or S4], □Murmur, □Muffled
    - *Grade:* □1–2[soft, only at PMI], □3–4[moderate, mild radiate], □5–6[loud, strong radiate, thrill]
    - *Timing:* □Systolic, □Diastolic, □Continuous
    - *PMI:*

	PMI	Over	Anatomic Boundaries
□	Lt. apex	Mitral valve	5th to 6th ICS at level of CCJ
□	Lt. base	Ao + Pul outflow	2nd to 4th ICS above the CCJ
□	Rt. midheart	Tricuspid valve	3rd to 5th ICS near the CCJ
□	Rt. sternal border	Right ventricle	5th to 7th ICS immediately dorsal to the sternum
□	Sternal (cat)	Sternum	In cats, determination of PMI offers very little clinical significance.

  - *Vertebral Heart Size:* Dog = 8.7–10.7; Cat = 6.9–8.1 (from cranial edge of T4)
  - *Innocent Murmur:* Grade 1-2, systolic, left base location, disappear by ~4 months of age, absent clinical signs

- **Pulses:**
  - *Pulse rate:*_____pulses/min
  - *Character:* □Sync, □Async; □Normokinetic, □Hyper-, □Hypo-, □Variable

- **Lungs:**
  - *Respiratory rate:*_____breaths/min [*RI*: 16–30]
  - *Depth/Effort:* □Norm, □Pant, □Deep, □Shallow, □↑ Insp. effort, □↑ Exp. effort
  - *Sounds/Localization:*
    - □Norm BV, □Quiet BV, □Loud BV, □Crack, □Wheez, □Frict, □Muffled
    - □All lung fields, □Rt cran, □Rt mid, □Rt caud, □Lt cran, □Lt mid, □Lt caud
  - *Tracheal Auscultation/ Palpation:* □Normal, Other:_____

- **Pain Score:**_____ / 5   Localization:_____

- **Mentation:** □BAR   □Confused/   □Drowsy/   □Stuporous   □Coma
  - □QAR   Disoriented   Obtunded   (unresponsive unless   (complete
  - □Dull   (conscious; inappropriate   (↓ interaction with   aroused by noxious   unresponsiveness
  - (conscious; responds   response to environment   environment; slow   stimuli)   to any stimuli)
  - to sensory stimuli)   [ex., vocalization, head   response to verbal
  -    pressing])   stimuli)

- **Skin Elasticity:** □Normal skin turgor, □↓ Skin turgor, □Skin tent, □Gelatinous

- **Mucus Membranes:**
  - *CRT:*_____ [*RI*: 1–2; <1 = compensated shock, sepsis, heat stroke; <2 = acute decompensated shock; >2 = late decompensated shock, decreased cardiac output, hypothermia]
  - *Color:*_____ [*RI*: pink; red = compensated shock, sepsis, heat stroke; pale/white = anemia, shock; blue = cyanosis; yellow = hepatic disease, extravascular hemolysis; brown = met-Hb]
  - *Texture:*_____ [*RI*: moist = hydrated; tacky-to-dry = 5–12% dehydrated]

Physical Exam – Systems Checklist:

- Head:_____ ☐NAF
  - Ears: ☐Ceruminous debris (mild / mod / sev) (AS / AD / AU), _____ ☐NAF
  - Eyes:_____ ☐NAF
    - Retinal:_____ ☐NAF

→ Ⓛ		Ⓡ		Ⓛ		Ⓡ ←	
☐	⊙ Normal Direct	☐	⊙ Normal Indirect	☐	⊙ Normal Indirect	☐	⊙ Normal Direct
☐	● Abnormal Direct	☐	● Abnormal Indirect	☐	● Abnormal Indirect	☐	● Abnormal Direct

  - Nose:_____ ☐NAF
  - Oral cavity: ☐Tarter/Gingivitis (mild / mod / sev), _____ ☐NAF
  - Mandibular lnn.: ☐Enlarged Lt., ☐Enlarged Rt., _____ ☐NAF

- Neck:_____ ☐NAF
  - Superficial cervical lnn.: ☐Enlarged Lt., ☐Enlarged Rt., _____ ☐NAF
  - Thyroid:_____ ☐NAF

- Thoracic limb:_____ ☐NAF
  - Foot pads:_____ ☐NAF
  - Knuckling:_____ ☐NAF
  - Axillary lnn. [normally absent]:_____ ☐NAF

- Thorax:_____ ☐NAF

- Abdomen:_____ ☐NAF
  - Mammary chain:_____ ☐NAF
  - Penis/ Testicles/ Vulva:_____ ☐NAF
  - Superficial inguinal lnn. [normally absent]:_____ ☐NAF

- Pelvic limb:_____ ☐NAF
  - Foot pads:_____ ☐NAF
  - Knuckling:_____ ☐NAF
  - Popliteal lnn.: ☐Enlarged Lt., ☐Enlarged Rt., _____ ☐NAF

- Skin:_____ ☐NAF
- Tail:_____ ☐NAF
- Rectal☞☉:_____ ☐NAF

Problems List:

- **Problem #1**:

- **Problem #2**:

- **Problem #3**:

- **Problem #4**:

- **Problem #5**:

- **Problem #6**:

Diagnostic Plan	Treatment Plan

Case No._____

Patient	Age	Sex		Breed	Weight
		nM	sF		
	DOB:	iM	iF	Color:	kg

Owner	Primary Veterinarian	Admit Date/ Time
Name: Phone:	Name: Phone:	Date: Time: AM / PM

• **Presenting complaint**:_____

_____

_____

_____

_____

• **Medical Hx**:_____

_____

_____

_____

_____

• **When/ where obtained**: Date:_____; ☐Breeder, ☐Shelter, Other:_____

Drug/ Supplement	Amount	Dose (mg/kg)	Route	Frequency	Date Started

• **Vaccine status – Dog**: ☐Rab ☐Parv ☐Dist ☐Aden; ☐Para ☐Lep ☐Bord ☐Influ ☐Lyme
• **Vaccine status – Cat**: ☐Rab ☐Herp ☐Cali ☐Pan ☐FeLV [kittens]; ☐FIV ☐Chlam ☐Bord
• **Heartworm / Flea & Tick / Intestinal Parasites**:
   ◦ *Last Heartworm Test*: Date:_____, ☐IDK; Test Results: ☐Pos, ☐Neg, ☐IDK
   ◦ *Monthly heartworm preventative*: ☐no ☐yes, Product:_____
   ◦ *Monthly flea & tick preventative*: ☐no ☐yes, Product:_____
   ◦ *Monthly dewormer*:   ☐no ☐yes, Product:_____
• **Surgical Hx**: ☐Spay/Neuter; Date:_____; Other:_____
• **Environment**: ☐Indoor, ☐Outdoor, Time spent outdoors/ Other:_____
• **Housemates**: Dogs:_____ Cats:_____ Other:_____
• **Diet**: ☐Wet, ☐Dry; Brand/ Amt.:_____

Appetite	☐Normal, ☐↑, ☐↓
Weight	☐Normal, ☐↑, ☐↓; Past Wt.:_____ kg; Date:_____; Δ:_____
Thirst	☐Normal, ☐↑, ☐↓
Urination	☐Normal, ☐↑, ☐↓, ☐Blood, ☐Strain
Defecation	☐Normal, ☐↑, ☐↓, ☐Blood, ☐Strain, ☐Diarrhea, ☐Mucus
Discharge	☐No, ☐Yes; Onset/ Describe:
Cough/ Sneeze	☐No, ☐Yes; Onset/ Describe:
Vomit	☐No, ☐Yes; Onset/ Describe:
Respiration	☐Normal, ☐↑ Rate, ☐↑ Effort
Energy level	☐Normal, ☐Lethargic, ☐Exercise intolerance

• **Travel Hx**: ☐None, Other:_____
• **Exposure to**: ☐Standing water, ☐Wildlife, ☐Board/daycare, ☐Dog park, ☐Groomer, ☐Pet store
• **Adverse reactions to food/ meds**: ☐None, Other:_____
• **Can give oral meds**: ☐no ☐yes; Helpful Tricks:_____

Physical Exam – General:

- **Body Weight**:_____kg **Body Condition Score**:___/9

- **Temperature**:_____°F [*Dog-RI*: 100.9–102.4; *Cat-RI*: 98.1–102.1]

- **Heart**:
  - *Rate*:_____beats/min [Dog-RI: 60–180; Cat-RI: 140–240 (in hospital)]
  - *Rhythm*: ☐Regular, ☐Irregular
  - *Sounds*: ☐None, ☐Split sound[S1 or S2], ☐Gallop[S3 or S4], ☐Murmur, ☐Muffled
    - *Grade*: ☐1–2[soft, only at PMI], ☐3–4[moderate, mild radiate], ☐5–6[loud, strong radiate, thrill]
    - *Timing*: ☐Systolic, ☐Diastolic, ☐Continuous
    - *PMI*:

	PMI	Over	Anatomic Boundaries
☐	Lt. apex	Mitral valve	5th to 6th ICS at level of CCJ
☐	Lt. base	Ao + Pul outflow	2nd to 4th ICS above the CCJ
☐	Rt. midheart	Tricuspid valve	3rd to 5th ICS near the CCJ
☐	Rt. sternal border	Right ventricle	5th to 7th ICS immediately dorsal to the sternum
☐	Sternal (cat)	Sternum	In cats, determination of PMI offers very little clinical significance.

  - *Vertebral Heart Size*: Dog = 8.7–10.7; Cat = 6.9–8.1 (from cranial edge of T4)
  - *Innocent Murmur*: Grade 1-2, systolic, left base location, disappear by ~4 months of age, absent clinical signs

- **Pulses**:
  - *Pulse rate*:_____pulses/min
  - *Character*: ☐Sync, ☐Async; ☐Normokinetic, ☐Hyper-, ☐Hypo-, ☐Variable

- **Lungs**:
  - *Respiratory rate*:_____breaths/min [*RI*: 16–30]
  - *Depth/Effort*: ☐Norm, ☐Pant, ☐Deep, ☐Shallow, ☐↑ Insp. effort, ☐↑ Exp. effort
  - *Sounds/Localization*:
    - ☐Norm BV, ☐Quiet BV, ☐Loud BV, ☐Crack, ☐Wheez, ☐Frict, ☐Muffled
    - ☐All lung fields, ☐Rt cran, ☐Rt mid, ☐Rt caud, ☐Lt cran, ☐Lt mid, ☐Lt caud
  - *Tracheal Auscultation/ Palpation*: ☐Normal, Other:_____

- **Pain Score**:_____ / 5   Localization:_____

- **Mentation**: ☐BAR   ☐Confused/   ☐Drowsy/   ☐Stuporous   ☐Coma
  ☐QAR   Disoriented   Obtunded   (unresponsive unless   (complete
  ☐Dull   (conscious; inappropriate   (↓ interaction with   aroused by noxious   unresponsiveness
  (conscious; responds   response to environment   environment; slow   stimuli)   to any stimuli)
  to sensory stimuli)   [ex., vocalization, head   response to verbal
  pressing])   stimuli)

- **Skin Elasticity**: ☐Normal skin turgor, ☐↓ Skin turgor, ☐Skin tent, ☐Gelatinous

- **Mucus Membranes**:
  - *CRT*:_____ [*RI*: 1–2; <1 = compensated shock, sepsis, heat stroke; <2 = acute decompensated shock;
    >2 = late decompensated shock, decreased cardiac output, hypothermia]
  - *Color*:_____ [*RI*: pink; red = compensated shock, sepsis, heat stroke; pale/white = anemia, shock;
    blue = cyanosis; yellow = hepatic disease, extravascular hemolysis; brown = met-Hb]
  - *Texture*:_____ [*RI*: moist = hydrated; tacky-to-dry = 5–12% dehydrated]

Physical Exam – Systems Checklist:

- Head: _____ ☐NAF
  - Ears: ☐Ceruminous debris (mild / mod / sev) (AS / AD / AU), _____ ☐NAF
  - Eyes: _____ ☐NAF
    - Retinal: _____ ☐NAF

→ Ⓛ		Ⓡ		Ⓛ		Ⓡ ←	
☐ ⊙ Normal Direct		☐ ⊙ Normal Indirect		☐ ⊙ Normal Indirect		☐ ⊙ Normal Direct	
☐ ⊙ Abnormal Direct		☐ ⊙ Abnormal Indirect		☐ ⊙ Abnormal Indirect		☐ ⊙ Abnormal Direct	

  - Nose: _____ ☐NAF
  - Oral cavity: ☐Tarter/Gingivitis (mild / mod / sev), _____ ☐NAF
  - Mandibular lnn.: ☐Enlarged Lt., ☐Enlarged Rt., _____ ☐NAF

- Neck: _____ ☐NAF
  - Superficial cervical lnn.: ☐Enlarged Lt., ☐Enlarged Rt., _____ ☐NAF
  - Thyroid: _____ ☐NAF

- Thoracic limb: _____ ☐NAF
  - Foot pads: _____ ☐NAF
  - Knuckling: _____ ☐NAF
  - Axillary lnn. [normally absent]: _____ ☐NAF

- Thorax: _____ ☐NAF

- Abdomen: _____ ☐NAF
  - Mammary chain: _____ ☐NAF
  - Penis/ Testicles/ Vulva: _____ ☐NAF
  - Superficial inguinal lnn. [normally absent]: _____ ☐NAF

- Pelvic limb: _____ ☐NAF
  - Foot pads: _____ ☐NAF
  - Knuckling: _____ ☐NAF
  - Popliteal lnn.: ☐Enlarged Lt., ☐Enlarged Rt., _____ ☐NAF

- Skin: _____ ☐NAF
- Tail: _____ ☐NAF
- Rectal☞⊙: _____ ☐NAF

Problems List:

- **Problem #1**:

- **Problem #2**:

- **Problem #3**:

- **Problem #4**:

- **Problem #5**:

- **Problem #6**:

Diagnostic Plan	Treatment Plan

Case No._____

Patient		Age		Sex		Breed		Weight
				nM	sF			
		DOB:		iM	iF	Color:		kg

Owner	Primary Veterinarian	Admit Date/ Time
Name: Phone:	Name: Phone:	Date: Time: AM / PM

• **Presenting complaint**:_____
_____
_____
_____
_____
_____

• **Medical Hx**:_____
_____
_____
_____
_____

• **When/ where obtained**: Date:_____; ☐Breeder, ☐Shelter, Other:_____

Drug/ Supplement	Amount	Dose (mg/kg)	Route	Frequency	Date Started

• **Vaccine status – Dog**: ☐Rab ☐Parv ☐Dist ☐Aden; ☐Para ☐Lep ☐Bord ☐Influ ☐Lyme
• **Vaccine status – Cat**: ☐Rab ☐Herp ☐Cali ☐Pan ☐FeLV [kittens]; ☐FIV ☐Chlam ☐Bord
• **Heartworm / Flea & Tick / Intestinal Parasites**:
  ◦ *Last Heartworm Test*: Date:_____, ☐IDK; Test Results: ☐Pos, ☐Neg, ☐IDK
  ◦ *Monthly heartworm preventative*: ☐no ☐yes, Product:_____
  ◦ *Monthly flea & tick preventative*: ☐no ☐yes, Product:_____
  ◦ *Monthly dewormer*:   ☐no ☐yes, Product:_____
• **Surgical Hx**: ☐Spay/Neuter; Date:_____; Other:_____
• **Environment**: ☐Indoor, ☐Outdoor, Time spent outdoors/ Other:_____
• **Housemates**: Dogs:_____ Cats:_____ Other:_____
• **Diet**: ☐Wet, ☐Dry; Brand/ Amt.:_____

Appetite	☐Normal, ☐↑, ☐↓
Weight	☐Normal, ☐↑, ☐↓; Past Wt.:_____ kg; Date:_____; Δ:_____
Thirst	☐Normal, ☐↑, ☐↓
Urination	☐Normal, ☐↑, ☐↓, ☐Blood, ☐Strain
Defecation	☐Normal, ☐↑, ☐↓, ☐Blood, ☐Strain, ☐Diarrhea, ☐Mucus
Discharge	☐No, ☐Yes; Onset/ Describe:
Cough/ Sneeze	☐No, ☐Yes; Onset/ Describe:
Vomit	☐No, ☐Yes; Onset/ Describe:
Respiration	☐Normal, ☐↑ Rate, ☐↑ Effort
Energy level	☐Normal, ☐Lethargic, ☐Exercise intolerance

• **Travel Hx**: ☐None, Other:_____
• **Exposure to**: ☐Standing water, ☐Wildlife, ☐Board/daycare, ☐Dog park, ☐Groomer, ☐Pet store
• **Adverse reactions to food/ meds**: ☐None, Other:_____
• **Can give oral meds**: ☐no ☐yes; Helpful Tricks:_____

Physical Exam – General:

- **Body Weight**:_____kg   **Body Condition Score**:___/9

- **Temperature**:_____°F [*Dog-RI*: 100.9–102.4; *Cat-RI*: 98.1–102.1]

- **Heart**:
  - *Rate*:_____beats/min [Dog-RI: 60–180; Cat-RI: 140–240 (in hospital)]
  - *Rhythm*: ☐Regular, ☐Irregular
  - *Sounds*: ☐None, ☐Split sound[S1 or S2], ☐Gallop[S3 or S4], ☐Murmur, ☐Muffled
    - *Grade*: ☐1–2[soft, only at PMI], ☐3–4[moderate, mild radiate], ☐5–6[loud, strong radiate, thrill]
    - *Timing*: ☐Systolic, ☐Diastolic, ☐Continuous
    - *PMI*:

	PMI	Over	Anatomic Boundaries
☐	Lt. apex	Mitral valve	5th to 6th ICS at level of CCJ
☐	Lt. base	Ao + Pul outflow	2nd to 4th ICS above the CCJ
☐	Rt. midheart	Tricuspid valve	3rd to 5th ICS near the CCJ
☐	Rt. sternal border	Right ventricle	5th to 7th ICS immediately dorsal to the sternum
☐	Sternal (cat)	Sternum	In cats, determination of PMI offers very little clinical significance.

  - • *Vertebral Heart Size*: Dog = 8.7–10.7; Cat = 6.9–8.1 (from cranial edge of T4)
  - • *Innocent Murmur*: Grade 1-2, systolic, left base location, disappear by ~4 months of age, absent clinical signs

- **Pulses**:
  - *Pulse rate*:_____pulses/min
  - *Character*: ☐Sync, ☐Async; ☐Normokinetic, ☐Hyper-, ☐Hypo-, ☐Variable

- **Lungs**:
  - *Respiratory rate*:_____breaths/min [*RI*: 16–30]
  - *Depth/Effort*: ☐Norm, ☐Pant, ☐Deep, ☐Shallow, ☐↑ Insp. effort, ☐↑ Exp. effort
  - *Sounds/Localization*:
    - ☐Norm BV, ☐Quiet BV, ☐Loud BV, ☐Crack, ☐Wheez, ☐Frict, ☐Muffled
    - ☐All lung fields, ☐Rt cran, ☐Rt mid, ☐Rt caud, ☐Lt cran, ☐Lt mid, ☐Lt caud
  - *Tracheal Auscultation/ Palpation*: ☐Normal, Other:_____

- **Pain Score**:_____ / 5   Localization:_____

- **Mentation**:

☐BAR ☐QAR ☐Dull (conscious; responds to sensory stimuli)	☐Confused/ Disoriented (conscious; inappropriate response to environment [ex., vocalization, head pressing])	☐Drowsy/ Obtunded (↓ interaction with environment; slow response to verbal stimuli)	☐Stuporous (unresponsive unless aroused by noxious stimuli)	☐Coma (complete unresponsiveness to any stimuli)

- **Skin Elasticity**: ☐Normal skin turgor, ☐↓ Skin turgor, ☐Skin tent, ☐Gelatinous

- **Mucus Membranes**:
  - *CRT*:_____ [*RI*: 1–2; <1 = compensated shock, sepsis, heat stroke; <2 = acute decompensated shock; >2 = late decompensated shock, decreased cardiac output, hypothermia]
  - *Color*:_____ [*RI*: pink; red = compensated shock, sepsis, heat stroke; pale/white = anemia, shock; blue = cyanosis; yellow = hepatic disease, extravascular hemolysis; brown = met-Hb]
  - *Texture*:_____ [*RI*: moist = hydrated; tacky-to-dry = 5–12% dehydrated]

Physical Exam – Systems Checklist:

- Head:_____ ☐NAF
  - ○ Ears: ☐Ceruminous debris (mild / mod / sev) (AS / AD / AU), _____ ☐NAF
  - ○ Eyes:_____ ☐NAF
    - ▪ Retinal:_____ ☐NAF

→ ⓛ	ⓡ	ⓛ	ⓡ ←
☐ ⊙ Normal Direct	☐ ⊙ Normal Indirect	☐ ⊙ Normal Indirect	☐ ⊙ Normal Direct
☐ ⊙ Abnormal Direct	☐ ⊙ Abnormal Indirect	☐ ⊙ Abnormal Indirect	☐ ⊙ Abnormal Direct

  - ○ Nose:_____ ☐NAF
  - ○ Oral cavity: ☐Tarter/Gingivitis (mild / mod / sev), _____ ☐NAF
  - ○ Mandibular lnn.: ☐Enlarged Lt., ☐Enlarged Rt., _____ ☐NAF

- Neck:_____ ☐NAF
  - ○ Superficial cervical lnn.: ☐Enlarged Lt., ☐Enlarged Rt., _____ ☐NAF
  - ○ Thyroid:_____ ☐NAF

- Thoracic limb:_____ ☐NAF
  - ○ Foot pads:_____ ☐NAF
  - ○ Knuckling:_____ ☐NAF
  - ○ Axillary lnn. [normally absent]:_____ ☐NAF

- Thorax:_____ ☐NAF

- Abdomen:_____ ☐NAF
  - ○ Mammary chain:_____ ☐NAF
  - ○ Penis/ Testicles/ Vulva:_____ ☐NAF
  - ○ Superficial inguinal lnn. [normally absent]:_____ ☐NAF

- Pelvic limb:_____ ☐NAF
  - ○ Foot pads:_____ ☐NAF
  - ○ Knuckling:_____ ☐NAF
  - ○ Popliteal lnn.: ☐Enlarged Lt., ☐Enlarged Rt., _____ ☐NAF

- Skin:_____ ☐NAF
- Tail:_____ ☐NAF
- Rectal☞⊙:_____ ☐NAF

Problems List:

- **Problem #1:**

- **Problem #2:**

- **Problem #3:**

- **Problem #4:**

- **Problem #5:**

- **Problem #6:**

Diagnostic Plan	Treatment Plan

Case No._____

Patient	Age	Sex		Breed	Weight
		nM	sF		
	DOB:	iM	iF	Color:	kg

Owner	Primary Veterinarian	Admit Date/ Time
Name: Phone:	Name: Phone:	Date: Time: AM / PM

• **Presenting complaint**:_____

_____

_____

_____

_____

_____

• **Medical Hx**:_____

_____

_____

_____

_____

• **When/ where obtained**: Date:_____; ☐Breeder, ☐Shelter, Other:_____

Drug/ Supplement	Amount	Dose (mg/kg)	Route	Frequency	Date Started

• **Vaccine status – Dog**: ☐Rab ☐Parv ☐Dist ☐Aden; ☐Para ☐Lep ☐Bord ☐Influ ☐Lyme
• **Vaccine status – Cat**: ☐Rab ☐Herp ☐Cali ☐Pan ☐FeLV [kittens]; ☐FIV ☐Chlam ☐Bord
• **Heartworm / Flea & Tick / Intestinal Parasites**:
  ◦ *Last Heartworm Test*: Date:_____, ☐IDK; Test Results: ☐Pos, ☐Neg, ☐IDK
  ◦ *Monthly heartworm preventative*: ☐no ☐yes, Product:_____
  ◦ *Monthly flea & tick preventative*: ☐no ☐yes, Product:_____
  ◦ *Monthly dewormer*: ☐no ☐yes, Product:_____
• **Surgical Hx**: ☐Spay/Neuter; Date:_____; Other:_____
• **Environment**: ☐Indoor, ☐Outdoor, Time spent outdoors/ Other:_____
• **Housemates**: Dogs:_____ Cats:_____ Other:_____
• **Diet**: ☐Wet, ☐Dry; Brand/ Amt.:_____

Appetite	☐Normal, ☐↑, ☐↓
Weight	☐Normal, ☐↑, ☐↓; Past Wt.:_____ kg; Date:_____; Δ:_____
Thirst	☐Normal, ☐↑, ☐↓
Urination	☐Normal, ☐↑, ☐↓, ☐Blood, ☐Strain
Defecation	☐Normal, ☐↑, ☐↓, ☐Blood, ☐Strain, ☐Diarrhea, ☐Mucus
Discharge	☐No, ☐Yes; Onset/ Describe:
Cough/ Sneeze	☐No, ☐Yes; Onset/ Describe:
Vomit	☐No, ☐Yes; Onset/ Describe:
Respiration	☐Normal, ☐↑ Rate, ☐↑ Effort
Energy level	☐Normal, ☐Lethargic, ☐Exercise intolerance

• **Travel Hx**: ☐None, Other:_____
• **Exposure to**: ☐Standing water, ☐Wildlife, ☐Board/daycare, ☐Dog park, ☐Groomer, ☐Pet store
• **Adverse reactions to food/ meds**: ☐None, Other:_____
• **Can give oral meds**: ☐no ☐yes; Helpful Tricks:_____

Physical Exam – General:

- **Body Weight:**_____kg   **Body Condition Score:**___/9

- **Temperature:**_____°F [*Dog-RI*: 100.9–102.4; *Cat-RI*: 98.1–102.1]

- **Heart:**
  - *Rate*:_____beats/min [Dog-RI: 60–180; Cat-RI: 140–240 (in hospital)]
  - *Rhythm*: ☐Regular, ☐Irregular
  - *Sounds*: ☐None, ☐Split sound[S1 or S2], ☐Gallop[S3 or S4], ☐Murmur, ☐Muffled
    - *Grade*: ☐1–2[soft, only at PMI],   ☐3–4[moderate, mild radiate],   ☐5–6[loud, strong radiate, thrill]
    - *Timing*: ☐Systolic, ☐Diastolic, ☐Continuous
    - *PMI*:

	PMI	Over	Anatomic Boundaries
☐	Lt. apex	Mitral valve	5th to 6th ICS at level of CCJ
☐	Lt. base	Ao + Pul outflow	2nd to 4th ICS above the CCJ
☐	Rt. midheart	Tricuspid valve	3rd to 5th ICS near the CCJ
☐	Rt. sternal border	Right ventricle	5th to 7th ICS immediately dorsal to the sternum
☐	Sternal (cat)	Sternum	In cats, determination of PMI offers very little clinical significance.

  - *Vertebral Heart Size*: Dog = 8.7–10.7; Cat = 6.9–8.1 (from cranial edge of T4)
  - *Innocent Murmur*: Grade 1-2, systolic, left base location, disappear by ~4 months of age, absent clinical signs

- **Pulses:**
  - *Pulse rate*:_____pulses/min
  - *Character*:   ☐Sync, ☐Async;   ☐Normokinetic, ☐Hyper-, ☐Hypo-, ☐Variable

- **Lungs:**
  - *Respiratory rate*:_____breaths/min [*RI*: 16–30]
  - *Depth/Effort*: ☐Norm, ☐Pant, ☐Deep, ☐Shallow, ☐↑ Insp. effort, ☐↑ Exp. effort
  - *Sounds/Localization*:
    - ☐Norm BV, ☐Quiet BV, ☐Loud BV, ☐Crack, ☐Wheez, ☐Frict, ☐Muffled
    - ☐All lung fields, ☐Rt cran, ☐Rt mid, ☐Rt caud, ☐Lt cran, ☐Lt mid, ☐Lt caud
  - *Tracheal Auscultation/ Palpation*: ☐Normal, Other:_____

- **Pain Score:**_____ / 5   Localization:_____

- **Mentation**: ☐BAR   ☐Confused/   ☐Drowsy/   ☐Stuporous   ☐Coma
  ☐QAR   Disoriented   Obtunded   (unresponsive unless   (complete
  ☐Dull   (conscious; inappropriate   (↓ interaction with   aroused by noxious   unresponsiveness
  (conscious; responds   response to environment   environment; slow   stimuli)   to any stimuli)
  to sensory stimuli)   [ex., vocalization, head   response to verbal
  pressing])   stimuli)

- **Skin Elasticity**: ☐Normal skin turgor, ☐↓ Skin turgor, ☐Skin tent, ☐Gelatinous

- **Mucus Membranes:**
  - *CRT*:_____ [*RI*: 1–2; <1 = compensated shock, sepsis, heat stroke; <2 = acute decompensated shock;
    >2 = late decompensated shock, decreased cardiac output, hypothermia]
  - *Color*:_____ [*RI*: pink; red = compensated shock, sepsis, heat stroke; pale/white = anemia, shock;
    blue = cyanosis; yellow = hepatic disease, extravascular hemolysis; brown = met-Hb]
  - *Texture*:_____ [*RI*: moist = hydrated; tacky-to-dry = 5–12% dehydrated]

Physical Exam – Systems Checklist:

- Head: _____ ☐NAF
  - Ears: ☐Ceruminous debris (mild / mod / sev) (AS / AD / AU), _____ ☐NAF
  - Eyes: _____ ☐NAF
    - Retinal: _____ ☐NAF

→ Ⓛ		Ⓡ		Ⓛ		Ⓡ ←	
☐ ⊙ Normal Direct		☐ ⊙ Normal Indirect		☐ ⊙ Normal Indirect		☐ ⊙ Normal Direct	
☐ ⦿ Abnormal Direct		☐ ⦿ Abnormal Indirect		☐ ⦿ Abnormal Indirect		☐ ⦿ Abnormal Direct	

  - Nose: _____ ☐NAF
  - Oral cavity: ☐Tarter/Gingivitis (mild / mod / sev), _____ ☐NAF
  - Mandibular lnn.: ☐Enlarged Lt., ☐Enlarged Rt., _____ ☐NAF

- Neck: _____ ☐NAF
  - Superficial cervical lnn.: ☐Enlarged Lt., ☐Enlarged Rt., _____ ☐NAF
  - Thyroid: _____ ☐NAF

- Thoracic limb: _____ ☐NAF
  - Foot pads: _____ ☐NAF
  - Knuckling: _____ ☐NAF
  - Axillary lnn. [normally absent]: _____ ☐NAF

- Thorax: _____ ☐NAF

- Abdomen: _____ ☐NAF
  - Mammary chain: _____ ☐NAF
  - Penis/ Testicles/ Vulva: _____ ☐NAF
  - Superficial inguinal lnn. [normally absent]: _____ ☐NAF

- Pelvic limb: _____ ☐NAF
  - Foot pads: _____ ☐NAF
  - Knuckling: _____ ☐NAF
  - Popliteal lnn.: ☐Enlarged Lt., ☐Enlarged Rt., _____ ☐NAF

- Skin: _____ ☐NAF
- Tail: _____ ☐NAF
- Rectal☞⊙: _____ ☐NAF

Problems List:

- **Problem #1**:

- **Problem #2**:

- **Problem #3**:

- **Problem #4**:

- **Problem #5**:

- **Problem #6**:

Diagnostic Plan	Treatment Plan

Case No._____

Patient	Age	Sex		Breed		Weight
		nM	sF			
	DOB:	iM	iF	Color:		kg

Owner	Primary Veterinarian	Admit Date/ Time
Name: Phone:	Name: Phone:	Date: Time: AM / PM

• **Presenting complaint**:_____
_____
_____
_____
_____
_____

• **Medical Hx**:_____
_____
_____
_____
_____

• **When/ where obtained**: Date:_____; ☐Breeder, ☐Shelter, Other:_____

Drug/ Supplement	Amount	Dose (mg/kg)	Route	Frequency	Date Started

• **Vaccine status – Dog**: ☐Rab ☐Parv ☐Dist ☐Aden; ☐Para ☐Lep ☐Bord ☐Influ ☐Lyme
• **Vaccine status – Cat**: ☐Rab ☐Herp ☐Cali ☐Pan ☐FeLV [kittens]; ☐FIV ☐Chlam ☐Bord
• **Heartworm / Flea & Tick / Intestinal Parasites**:
   ◦ *Last Heartworm Test*: Date:_____, ☐IDK; Test Results: ☐Pos, ☐Neg, ☐IDK
   ◦ *Monthly heartworm preventative*: ☐no ☐yes, Product:_____
   ◦ *Monthly flea & tick preventative*: ☐no ☐yes, Product:_____
   ◦ *Monthly dewormer*:   ☐no ☐yes, Product:_____
• **Surgical Hx**: ☐Spay/Neuter; Date:_____; Other:_____
• **Environment**: ☐Indoor, ☐Outdoor, Time spent outdoors/ Other:_____
• **Housemates**: Dogs:_____ Cats:_____ Other:_____
• **Diet**: ☐Wet, ☐Dry; Brand/ Amt.:_____

Appetite	☐Normal, ☐↑, ☐↓
Weight	☐Normal, ☐↑, ☐↓; Past Wt.:_____ kg; Date:_____; Δ:_____
Thirst	☐Normal, ☐↑, ☐↓
Urination	☐Normal, ☐↑, ☐↓, ☐Blood, ☐Strain
Defecation	☐Normal, ☐↑, ☐↓, ☐Blood, ☐Strain, ☐Diarrhea, ☐Mucus
Discharge	☐No, ☐Yes; Onset/ Describe:
Cough/ Sneeze	☐No, ☐Yes; Onset/ Describe:
Vomit	☐No, ☐Yes; Onset/ Describe:
Respiration	☐Normal, ☐↑ Rate, ☐↑ Effort
Energy level	☐Normal, ☐Lethargic, ☐Exercise intolerance

• **Travel Hx**: ☐None, Other:_____
• **Exposure to**: ☐Standing water, ☐Wildlife, ☐Board/daycare, ☐Dog park, ☐Groomer, ☐Pet store
• **Adverse reactions to food/ meds**: ☐None, Other:_____
• **Can give oral meds**: ☐no ☐yes; Helpful Tricks:_____

Physical Exam – General:

- **Body Weight**:_____kg   **Body Condition Score**:___/9

- **Temperature**:_____°F [*Dog-RI*: 100.9–102.4; *Cat-RI*: 98.1–102.1]

- **Heart**:
  - *Rate*:_____beats/min [Dog-RI: 60–180; Cat-RI: 140–240 (in hospital)]
  - *Rhythm*: ☐Regular, ☐Irregular
  - *Sounds*: ☐None, ☐Split sound[S1 or S2], ☐Gallop[S3 or S4], ☐Murmur, ☐Muffled
    - *Grade*: ☐1–2[soft, only at PMI], ☐3–4[moderate, mild radiate], ☐5–6[loud, strong radiate, thrill]
    - *Timing*: ☐Systolic, ☐Diastolic, ☐Continuous
    - *PMI*:

	PMI	Over	Anatomic Boundaries
☐	Lt. apex	Mitral valve	5th to 6th ICS at level of CCJ
☐	Lt. base	Ao + Pul outflow	2nd to 4th ICS above the CCJ
☐	Rt. midheart	Tricuspid valve	3rd to 5th ICS near the CCJ
☐	Rt. sternal border	Right ventricle	5th to 7th ICS immediately dorsal to the sternum
☐	Sternal (cat)	Sternum	In cats, determination of PMI offers very little clinical significance.

  - • *Vertebral Heart Size*: Dog = 8.7–10.7; Cat = 6.9–8.1 (from cranial edge of T4)
  - • *Innocent Murmur*: Grade 1-2, systolic, left base location, disappear by ~4 months of age, absent clinical signs

- **Pulses**:
  - *Pulse rate*:_____pulses/min
  - *Character*: ☐Sync, ☐Async; ☐Normokinetic, ☐Hyper-, ☐Hypo-, ☐Variable

- **Lungs**:
  - *Respiratory rate*:_____breaths/min [*RI*: 16–30]
  - *Depth/Effort*: ☐Norm, ☐Pant, ☐Deep, ☐Shallow, ☐↑ Insp. effort, ☐↑ Exp. effort
  - *Sounds/Localization*:
    - ☐Norm BV, ☐Quiet BV, ☐Loud BV, ☐Crack, ☐Wheez, ☐Frict, ☐Muffled
    - ☐All lung fields, ☐Rt cran, ☐Rt mid, ☐Rt caud, ☐Lt cran, ☐Lt mid, ☐Lt caud
  - *Tracheal Auscultation/ Palpation*: ☐Normal, Other:_____

- **Pain Score**:_____ / 5   Localization:_____

- **Mentation**:

☐BAR ☐QAR ☐Dull (conscious; responds to sensory stimuli)	☐Confused/ Disoriented (conscious; inappropriate response to environment [ex., vocalization, head pressing])	☐Drowsy/ Obtunded (↓ interaction with environment; slow response to verbal stimuli)	☐Stuporous (unresponsive unless aroused by noxious stimuli)	☐Coma (complete unresponsiveness to any stimuli)

- **Skin Elasticity**: ☐Normal skin turgor, ☐↓ Skin turgor, ☐Skin tent, ☐Gelatinous

- **Mucus Membranes**:
  - *CRT*:_____ [*RI*: 1–2; <1 = compensated shock, sepsis, heat stroke; <2 = acute decompensated shock; >2 = late decompensated shock, decreased cardiac output, hypothermia]
  - *Color*:_____ [*RI*: pink; red = compensated shock, sepsis, heat stroke; pale/white = anemia, shock; blue = cyanosis; yellow = hepatic disease, extravascular hemolysis; brown = met-Hb]
  - *Texture*:_____ [*RI*: moist = hydrated; tacky-to-dry = 5–12% dehydrated]

Physical Exam – Systems Checklist:

- Head: _____ ☐NAF
  - Ears: ☐Ceruminous debris (mild / mod / sev) (AS / AD / AU), _____ ☐NAF
  - Eyes: _____ ☐NAF
    - Retinal: _____ ☐NAF

→ Ⓛ		Ⓡ		Ⓛ		Ⓡ ←	
☐	⊙ Normal Direct	☐	⊙ Normal Indirect	☐	⊙ Normal Indirect	☐	⊙ Normal Direct
☐	◉ Abnormal Direct	☐	◉ Abnormal Indirect	☐	◉ Abnormal Indirect	☐	◉ Abnormal Direct

  - Nose: _____ ☐NAF
  - Oral cavity: ☐Tarter/Gingivitis (mild / mod / sev), _____ ☐NAF
  - Mandibular lnn.: ☐Enlarged Lt., ☐Enlarged Rt., _____ ☐NAF

- Neck: _____ ☐NAF
  - Superficial cervical lnn.: ☐Enlarged Lt., ☐Enlarged Rt., _____ ☐NAF
  - Thyroid: _____ ☐NAF

- Thoracic limb: _____ ☐NAF
  - Foot pads: _____ ☐NAF
  - Knuckling: _____ ☐NAF
  - Axillary lnn. [normally absent]: _____ ☐NAF

- Thorax: _____ ☐NAF

- Abdomen: _____ ☐NAF
  - Mammary chain: _____ ☐NAF
  - Penis/ Testicles/ Vulva: _____ ☐NAF
  - Superficial inguinal lnn. [normally absent]: _____ ☐NAF

- Pelvic limb: _____ ☐NAF
  - Foot pads: _____ ☐NAF
  - Knuckling: _____ ☐NAF
  - Popliteal lnn.: ☐Enlarged Lt., ☐Enlarged Rt., _____ ☐NAF

- Skin: _____ ☐NAF
- Tail: _____ ☐NAF
- Rectal☞⊙: _____ ☐NAF

Problems List:

- **Problem #1**:

- **Problem #2**:

- **Problem #3**:

- **Problem #4**:

- **Problem #5**:

- **Problem #6**:

Diagnostic Plan	Treatment Plan

Case No._____

Patient	Age	Sex		Breed	Weight
		nM	sF		
	DOB:	iM	iF	Color:	kg

Owner		Primary Veterinarian	Admit Date/ Time
Name: Phone:		Name: Phone:	Date: Time: AM / PM

• **Presenting complaint**:_____

_____

_____

_____

_____

• **Medical Hx**:_____

_____

_____

_____

_____

• **When/ where obtained**: Date:_____; □Breeder, □Shelter, Other:_____

Drug/ Supplement	Amount	Dose (mg/kg)	Route	Frequency	Date Started

• **Vaccine status – Dog**: □Rab □Parv □Dist □Aden; □Para □Lep □Bord □Influ □Lyme
• **Vaccine status – Cat**: □Rab □Herp □Cali □Pan □FeLV [kittens]; □FIV □Chlam □Bord
• **Heartworm / Flea & Tick / Intestinal Parasites**:
  ◦ *Last Heartworm Test*: Date:_____, □IDK; Test Results: □Pos, □Neg, □IDK
  ◦ *Monthly heartworm preventative*: □no □yes, Product:_____
  ◦ *Monthly flea & tick preventative*: □no □yes, Product:_____
  ◦ *Monthly dewormer*: □no □yes, Product:_____
• **Surgical Hx**: □Spay/Neuter; Date:_____; Other:_____
• **Environment**: □Indoor, □Outdoor, Time spent outdoors/ Other:_____
• **Housemates**: Dogs:_____ Cats:_____ Other:_____
• **Diet**: □Wet, □Dry; Brand/ Amt.:_____

Appetite	□Normal, □↑, □↓
Weight	□Normal, □↑, □↓; Past Wt.:_____ kg; Date:_____; Δ:_____
Thirst	□Normal, □↑, □↓
Urination	□Normal, □↑, □↓, □Blood, □Strain
Defecation	□Normal, □↑, □↓, □Blood, □Strain, □Diarrhea, □Mucus
Discharge	□No, □Yes; Onset/ Describe:
Cough/ Sneeze	□No, □Yes; Onset/ Describe:
Vomit	□No, □Yes; Onset/ Describe:
Respiration	□Normal, □↑ Rate, □↑ Effort
Energy level	□Normal, □Lethargic, □Exercise intolerance

• **Travel Hx**: □None, Other:_____
• **Exposure to**: □Standing water, □Wildlife, □Board/daycare, □Dog park, □Groomer, □Pet store
• **Adverse reactions to food/ meds**: □None, Other:_____
• **Can give oral meds**: □no □yes; Helpful Tricks:_____

Physical Exam – General:

• **Body Weight**:_____kg   **Body Condition Score**:____/9

• **Temperature**:_____°F [*Dog-RI*: 100.9–102.4; *Cat-RI*: 98.1–102.1]

• **Heart**:
  ◦ *Rate*:_____beats/min [Dog-RI: 60–180; Cat-RI: 140–240 (in hospital)]
  ◦ *Rhythm*: ☐Regular, ☐Irregular
  ◦ *Sounds*: ☐None, ☐Split sound[S1 or S2], ☐Gallop[S3 or S4], ☐Murmur, ☐Muffled
    ▪ *Grade*: ☐1–2[soft, only at PMI], ☐3–4[moderate, mild radiate], ☐5–6[loud, strong radiate, thrill]
    ▪ *Timing*: ☐Systolic, ☐Diastolic, ☐Continuous
    ▪ *PMI*:

	PMI	Over	Anatomic Boundaries
☐	Lt. apex	Mitral valve	5th to 6th ICS at level of CCJ
☐	Lt. base	Ao + Pul outflow	2nd to 4th ICS above the CCJ
☐	Rt. midheart	Tricuspid valve	3rd to 5th ICS near the CCJ
☐	Rt. sternal border	Right ventricle	5th to 7th ICS immediately dorsal to the sternum
☐	Sternal (cat)	Sternum	In cats, determination of PMI offers very little clinical significance.

  • *Vertebral Heart Size*: Dog = 8.7–10.7; Cat = 6.9–8.1 (from cranial edge of T4)
  • *Innocent Murmur*: Grade 1-2, systolic, left base location, disappear by ~4 months of age, absent clinical signs

• **Pulses**:
  ◦ *Pulse rate*:_____pulses/min
  ◦ *Character*: ☐Sync, ☐Async; ☐Normokinetic, ☐Hyper-, ☐Hypo-, ☐Variable

• **Lungs**:
  ◦ *Respiratory rate*:_____breaths/min [*RI*: 16–30]
  ◦ *Depth/Effort*: ☐Norm, ☐Pant, ☐Deep, ☐Shallow, ☐↑ Insp. effort, ☐↑ Exp. effort
  ◦ *Sounds/Localization*:
    ▪ ☐Norm BV, ☐Quiet BV, ☐Loud BV, ☐Crack, ☐Wheez, ☐Frict, ☐Muffled
    ▪ ☐All lung fields, ☐Rt cran, ☐Rt mid, ☐Rt caud, ☐Lt cran, ☐Lt mid, ☐Lt caud
  ◦ *Tracheal Auscultation/ Palpation*: ☐Normal, Other:_____

• **Pain Score**:_____ / 5   Localization:_____

• **Mentation**:
  ☐BAR / ☐QAR / ☐Dull (conscious; responds to sensory stimuli)
  ☐Confused/ Disoriented (conscious; inappropriate response to environment [ex., vocalization, head pressing])
  ☐Drowsy/ Obtunded (↓ interaction with environment; slow response to verbal stimuli)
  ☐Stuporous (unresponsive unless aroused by noxious stimuli)
  ☐Coma (complete unresponsiveness to any stimuli)

• **Skin Elasticity**: ☐Normal skin turgor, ☐↓ Skin turgor, ☐Skin tent, ☐Gelatinous

• **Mucus Membranes**:
  ◦ *CRT*:_____ [*RI*: 1–2; <1 = compensated shock, sepsis, heat stroke; <2 = acute decompensated shock; >2 = late decompensated shock, decreased cardiac output, hypothermia]
  ◦ *Color*:_____ [*RI*: pink; red = compensated shock, sepsis, heat stroke; pale/white = anemia, shock; blue = cyanosis; yellow = hepatic disease, extravascular hemolysis; brown = met-Hb]
  ◦ *Texture*:_____ [*RI*: moist = hydrated; tacky-to-dry = 5–12% dehydrated]

Physical Exam – Systems Checklist:

- Head: _____ ☐NAF
  - Ears: ☐Ceruminous debris (mild / mod / sev) (AS / AD / AU), _____ ☐NAF
  - Eyes: _____ ☐NAF
    - Retinal: _____ ☐NAF

→ ⓛ		ⓡ		ⓛ		ⓡ ←	
☐	⊙ Normal Direct	☐	⊙ Normal Indirect	☐	⊙ Normal Indirect	☐	⊙ Normal Direct
☐	● Abnormal Direct	☐	● Abnormal Indirect	☐	● Abnormal Indirect	☐	● Abnormal Direct

  - Nose: _____ ☐NAF
  - Oral cavity: ☐Tarter/Gingivitis (mild / mod / sev), _____ ☐NAF
  - Mandibular lnn.: ☐Enlarged Lt., ☐Enlarged Rt., _____ ☐NAF

- Neck: _____ ☐NAF
  - Superficial cervical lnn.: ☐Enlarged Lt., ☐Enlarged Rt., _____ ☐NAF
  - Thyroid: _____ ☐NAF

- Thoracic limb: _____ ☐NAF
  - Foot pads: _____ ☐NAF
  - Knuckling: _____ ☐NAF
  - Axillary lnn. [normally absent]: _____ ☐NAF

- Thorax: _____ ☐NAF

- Abdomen: _____ ☐NAF
  - Mammary chain: _____ ☐NAF
  - Penis/ Testicles/ Vulva: _____ ☐NAF
  - Superficial inguinal lnn. [normally absent]: _____ ☐NAF

- Pelvic limb: _____ ☐NAF
  - Foot pads: _____ ☐NAF
  - Knuckling: _____ ☐NAF
  - Popliteal lnn.: ☐Enlarged Lt., ☐Enlarged Rt., _____ ☐NAF

- Skin: _____ ☐NAF
- Tail: _____ ☐NAF
- Rectal☞☉: _____ ☐NAF

Problems List:

- **Problem #1:**

- **Problem #2:**

- **Problem #3:**

- **Problem #4:**

- **Problem #5:**

- **Problem #6:**

Diagnostic Plan	Treatment Plan

Case No._____

Patient	Age	Sex		Breed	Weight
		nM	sF		kg
	DOB:	iM	iF	Color:	

Owner	Primary Veterinarian	Admit Date/ Time
Name: Phone:	Name: Phone:	Date: Time: AM / PM

• **Presenting complaint**:_____
_____
_____
_____
_____
_____

• **Medical Hx**:_____
_____
_____
_____
_____

• **When/ where obtained**: Date:_____; ☐Breeder, ☐Shelter, Other:_____

Drug/ Supplement	Amount	Dose (mg/kg)	Route	Frequency	Date Started

• **Vaccine status – Dog**: ☐Rab ☐Parv ☐Dist ☐Aden; ☐Para ☐Lep ☐Bord ☐Influ ☐Lyme
• **Vaccine status – Cat**: ☐Rab ☐Herp ☐Cali ☐Pan ☐FeLV [kittens]; ☐FIV ☐Chlam ☐Bord
• **Heartworm / Flea & Tick / Intestinal Parasites**:
  ◦ *Last Heartworm Test*: Date:_____, ☐IDK; Test Results: ☐Pos, ☐Neg, ☐IDK
  ◦ *Monthly heartworm preventative*: ☐no ☐yes, Product:_____
  ◦ *Monthly flea & tick preventative*: ☐no ☐yes, Product:_____
  ◦ *Monthly dewormer*:   ☐no ☐yes, Product:_____
• **Surgical Hx**: ☐Spay/Neuter; Date:_____; Other:_____
• **Environment**: ☐Indoor, ☐Outdoor, Time spent outdoors/ Other:_____
• **Housemates**: Dogs:_____ Cats:_____ Other:_____
• **Diet**: ☐Wet, ☐Dry; Brand/ Amt.:_____

Appetite	☐Normal, ☐↑, ☐↓
Weight	☐Normal, ☐↑, ☐↓; Past Wt.:_____ kg; Date:_____; Δ:_____
Thirst	☐Normal, ☐↑, ☐↓
Urination	☐Normal, ☐↑, ☐↓, ☐Blood, ☐Strain
Defecation	☐Normal, ☐↑, ☐↓, ☐Blood, ☐Strain, ☐Diarrhea, ☐Mucus
Discharge	☐No, ☐Yes; Onset/ Describe:
Cough/ Sneeze	☐No, ☐Yes; Onset/ Describe:
Vomit	☐No, ☐Yes; Onset/ Describe:
Respiration	☐Normal, ☐↑ Rate, ☐↑ Effort
Energy level	☐Normal, ☐Lethargic, ☐Exercise intolerance

• **Travel Hx**: ☐None, Other:_____
• **Exposure to**: ☐Standing water, ☐Wildlife, ☐Board/daycare, ☐Dog park, ☐Groomer, ☐Pet store
• **Adverse reactions to food/ meds**: ☐None, Other:_____
• **Can give oral meds**: ☐no ☐yes; Helpful Tricks:_____

Physical Exam – General:

- **Body Weight**:_____kg   **Body Condition Score**:___/9

- **Temperature**:_____°F [*Dog-RI*: 100.9–102.4;   *Cat-RI*: 98.1–102.1]

- **Heart**:
  - *Rate*:_____beats/min [Dog-RI: 60–180;   Cat-RI: 140–240 (in hospital)]
  - *Rhythm*: ☐Regular, ☐Irregular
  - *Sounds*:   ☐None, ☐Split sound[S1 or S2], ☐Gallop[S3 or S4], ☐Murmur, ☐Muffled
    - *Grade*:   ☐1–2[soft, only at PMI],   ☐3–4[moderate, mild radiate],   ☐5–6[loud, strong radiate, thrill]
    - *Timing*: ☐Systolic, ☐Diastolic, ☐Continuous
    - *PMI*:

	PMI	Over	Anatomic Boundaries
☐	Lt. apex	Mitral valve	5th to 6th ICS at level of CCJ
☐	Lt. base	Ao + Pul outflow	2nd to 4th ICS above the CCJ
☐	Rt. midheart	Tricuspid valve	3rd to 5th ICS near the CCJ
☐	Rt. sternal border	Right ventricle	5th to 7th ICS immediately dorsal to the sternum
☐	Sternal (cat)	Sternum	In cats, determination of PMI offers very little clinical significance.

  - •   *Vertebral Heart Size*: Dog = 8.7–10.7; Cat = 6.9–8.1 (from cranial edge of T4)
  - •   *Innocent Murmur*: Grade 1-2, systolic, left base location, disappear by ~4 months of age, absent clinical signs

- **Pulses**:
  - *Pulse rate*:_____pulses/min
  - *Character*:   ☐Sync, ☐Async;   ☐Normokinetic, ☐Hyper-, ☐Hypo-, ☐Variable

- **Lungs**:
  - *Respiratory rate*:_____breaths/min [*RI*: 16–30]
  - *Depth/Effort*: ☐Norm, ☐Pant, ☐Deep, ☐Shallow, ☐↑ Insp. effort, ☐↑ Exp. effort
  - *Sounds/Localization*:
    - ☐Norm BV, ☐Quiet BV, ☐Loud BV, ☐Crack, ☐Wheez, ☐Frict, ☐Muffled
    - ☐All lung fields, ☐Rt cran, ☐Rt mid, ☐Rt caud, ☐Lt cran, ☐Lt mid, ☐Lt caud
  - *Tracheal Auscultation/ Palpation*: ☐Normal, Other:_____

- **Pain Score**:_____ / 5   Localization:_____

- **Mentation**:

☐BAR ☐QAR ☐Dull (conscious; responds to sensory stimuli)	☐Confused/ Disoriented (conscious; inappropriate response to environment [ex., vocalization, head pressing])	☐Drowsy/ Obtunded (↓ interaction with environment; slow response to verbal stimuli)	☐Stuporous (unresponsive unless aroused by noxious stimuli)	☐Coma (complete unresponsiveness to any stimuli)

- **Skin Elasticity**: ☐Normal skin turgor, ☐↓ Skin turgor, ☐Skin tent, ☐Gelatinous

- **Mucus Membranes**:
  - *CRT*:_____ [*RI*: 1–2; <1 = compensated shock, sepsis, heat stroke; <2 = acute decompensated shock; >2 = late decompensated shock, decreased cardiac output, hypothermia]
  - *Color*:_____ [*RI*: pink; red = compensated shock, sepsis, heat stroke; pale/white = anemia, shock; blue = cyanosis; yellow = hepatic disease, extravascular hemolysis; brown = met-Hb]
  - *Texture*:_____ [*RI*: moist = hydrated; tacky-to-dry = 5–12% dehydrated]

Physical Exam – Systems Checklist:

- Head: _____ ☐NAF
  - Ears: ☐Ceruminous debris (mild / mod / sev) (AS / AD / AU), _____ ☐NAF
  - Eyes: _____ ☐NAF
    - Retinal: _____ ☐NAF

→ ⑬		⑱		⑬		⑱ ←	
☐	⊙ Normal Direct	☐	⊙ Normal Indirect	☐	⊙ Normal Indirect	☐	⊙ Normal Direct
☐	⦿ Abnormal Direct	☐	⦿ Abnormal Indirect	☐	⦿ Abnormal Indirect	☐	⦿ Abnormal Direct

  - Nose: _____ ☐NAF
  - Oral cavity: ☐Tarter/Gingivitis (mild / mod / sev), _____ ☐NAF
  - Mandibular lnn.: ☐Enlarged Lt., ☐Enlarged Rt., _____ ☐NAF

- Neck: _____ ☐NAF
  - Superficial cervical lnn.: ☐Enlarged Lt., ☐Enlarged Rt., _____ ☐NAF
  - Thyroid: _____ ☐NAF

- Thoracic limb: _____ ☐NAF
  - Foot pads: _____ ☐NAF
  - Knuckling: _____ ☐NAF
  - Axillary lnn. [normally absent]: _____ ☐NAF

- Thorax: _____ ☐NAF

- Abdomen: _____ ☐NAF
  - Mammary chain: _____ ☐NAF
  - Penis/ Testicles/ Vulva: _____ ☐NAF
  - Superficial inguinal lnn. [normally absent]: _____ ☐NAF

- Pelvic limb: _____ ☐NAF
  - Foot pads: _____ ☐NAF
  - Knuckling: _____ ☐NAF
  - Popliteal lnn.: ☐Enlarged Lt., ☐Enlarged Rt., _____ ☐NAF

- Skin: _____ ☐NAF
- Tail: _____ ☐NAF
- Rectal ☞ ☉: _____ ☐NAF

Problems List:

• **Problem #1**:

• **Problem #2**:

• **Problem #3**:

• **Problem #4**:

• **Problem #5**:

• **Problem #6**:

Diagnostic Plan	Treatment Plan

Case No._____

Patient	Age	Sex		Breed	Weight
		nM	sF		
	DOB:	iM	iF	Color:	kg

Owner	Primary Veterinarian	Admit Date/ Time
Name: Phone:	Name: Phone:	Date: Time: AM / PM

• **Presenting complaint**:_____
_____
_____
_____
_____
_____

• **Medical Hx**:_____
_____
_____
_____
_____
_____

• **When/ where obtained**: Date:_____; □Breeder, □Shelter, Other:_____

Drug/ Supplement	Amount	Dose (mg/kg)	Route	Frequency	Date Started

• **Vaccine status – Dog**: □Rab □Parv □Dist □Aden; □Para □Lep □Bord □Influ □Lyme
• **Vaccine status – Cat**: □Rab □Herp □Cali □Pan □FeLV [kittens]; □FIV □Chlam □Bord
• **Heartworm / Flea & Tick / Intestinal Parasites**:
  ◦ *Last Heartworm Test*: Date:_____, □IDK; Test Results: □Pos, □Neg, □IDK
  ◦ *Monthly heartworm preventative*: □no □yes, Product:_____
  ◦ *Monthly flea & tick preventative*: □no □yes, Product:_____
  ◦ *Monthly dewormer*: □no □yes, Product:_____
• **Surgical Hx**: □Spay/Neuter; Date:_____; Other:_____
• **Environment**: □Indoor, □Outdoor, Time spent outdoors/ Other:_____
• **Housemates**: Dogs:_____ Cats:_____ Other:_____
• **Diet**: □Wet, □Dry; Brand/ Amt.:_____

Appetite	□Normal, □↑, □↓
Weight	□Normal, □↑, □↓; Past Wt.:_____ kg; Date:_____; Δ:_____
Thirst	□Normal, □↑, □↓
Urination	□Normal, □↑, □↓, □Blood, □Strain
Defecation	□Normal, □↑, □↓, □Blood, □Strain, □Diarrhea, □Mucus
Discharge	□No, □Yes; Onset/ Describe:
Cough/ Sneeze	□No, □Yes; Onset/ Describe:
Vomit	□No, □Yes; Onset/ Describe:
Respiration	□Normal, □↑ Rate, □↑ Effort
Energy level	□Normal, □Lethargic, □Exercise intolerance

• **Travel Hx**: □None, Other:_____
• **Exposure to**: □Standing water, □Wildlife, □Board/daycare, □Dog park, □Groomer, □Pet store
• **Adverse reactions to food/ meds**: □None, Other:_____
• **Can give oral meds**: □no □yes; Helpful Tricks:_____

Physical Exam – General:

- **Body Weight**:_____kg   **Body Condition Score**:___/9

- **Temperature**:_____°F [*Dog-RI*: 100.9–102.4; *Cat-RI*: 98.1–102.1]

- **Heart**:
  - *Rate*:_____beats/min [Dog-RI: 60–180; Cat-RI: 140–240 (in hospital)]
  - *Rhythm*: ☐Regular, ☐Irregular
  - *Sounds*: ☐None, ☐Split sound[S1 or S2], ☐Gallop[S3 or S4], ☐Murmur, ☐Muffled
    - *Grade*: ☐1–2[soft, only at PMI],   ☐3–4[moderate, mild radiate],   ☐5–6[loud, strong radiate, thrill]
    - *Timing*: ☐Systolic, ☐Diastolic, ☐Continuous
    - *PMI*:

	PMI	Over	Anatomic Boundaries
☐	Lt. apex	Mitral valve	5th to 6th ICS at level of CCJ
☐	Lt. base	Ao + Pul outflow	2nd to 4th ICS above the CCJ
☐	Rt. midheart	Tricuspid valve	3rd to 5th ICS near the CCJ
☐	Rt. sternal border	Right ventricle	5th to 7th ICS immediately dorsal to the sternum
☐	Sternal (cat)	Sternum	In cats, determination of PMI offers very little clinical significance.

  - *Vertebral Heart Size*: Dog = 8.7–10.7; Cat = 6.9–8.1 (from cranial edge of T4)
  - *Innocent Murmur*: Grade 1-2, systolic, left base location, disappear by ~4 months of age, absent clinical signs

- **Pulses**:
  - *Pulse rate*:_____pulses/min
  - *Character*:   ☐Sync, ☐Async;   ☐Normokinetic, ☐Hyper-, ☐Hypo-, ☐Variable

- **Lungs**:
  - *Respiratory rate*:_____breaths/min [*RI*: 16–30]
  - *Depth/Effort*: ☐Norm, ☐Pant, ☐Deep, ☐Shallow, ☐↑ Insp. effort, ☐↑ Exp. effort
  - *Sounds/Localization*:
    - ☐Norm BV, ☐Quiet BV, ☐Loud BV, ☐Crack, ☐Wheez, ☐Frict, ☐Muffled
    - ☐All lung fields, ☐Rt cran, ☐Rt mid, ☐Rt caud, ☐Lt cran, ☐Lt mid, ☐Lt caud
  - *Tracheal Auscultation/ Palpation*: ☐Normal, Other:_____

- **Pain Score**:_____ / 5   Localization:_____

- **Mentation**:

☐BAR	☐Confused/	☐Drowsy/	☐Stuporous	☐Coma
☐QAR	Disoriented	Obtunded	(unresponsive unless aroused by noxious stimuli)	(complete unresponsiveness to any stimuli)
☐Dull	(conscious; inappropriate response to environment [ex., vocalization, head pressing])	(↓ interaction with environment; slow response to verbal stimuli)		
(conscious; responds to sensory stimuli)				

- **Skin Elasticity**: ☐Normal skin turgor, ☐↓ Skin turgor, ☐Skin tent, ☐Gelatinous

- **Mucus Membranes**:
  - *CRT*:_____ [*RI*: 1–2; <1 = compensated shock, sepsis, heat stroke; <2 = acute decompensated shock; >2 = late decompensated shock, decreased cardiac output, hypothermia]
  - *Color*:_____ [*RI*: pink; red = compensated shock, sepsis, heat stroke; pale/white = anemia, shock; blue = cyanosis; yellow = hepatic disease, extravascular hemolysis; brown = met-Hb]
  - *Texture*:_____ [*RI*: moist = hydrated; tacky-to-dry = 5–12% dehydrated]

Physical Exam – Systems Checklist:

- Head:_____ ☐NAF
  - Ears: ☐Ceruminous debris (mild / mod / sev) (AS / AD / AU), _____ ☐NAF
  - Eyes:_____ ☐NAF
    - Retinal:_____ ☐NAF

→ Ⓛ		Ⓡ		Ⓛ		Ⓡ ←	
☐ ⊙ Normal Direct		☐ ⊙ Normal Indirect		☐ ⊙ Normal Indirect		☐ ⊙ Normal Direct	
☐ ⊙ Abnormal Direct		☐ ⊙ Abnormal Indirect		☐ ⊙ Abnormal Indirect		☐ ⊙ Abnormal Direct	

  - Nose:_____ ☐NAF
  - Oral cavity: ☐Tarter/Gingivitis (mild / mod / sev), _____ ☐NAF
  - Mandibular lnn.: ☐Enlarged Lt., ☐Enlarged Rt., _____ ☐NAF

- Neck:_____ ☐NAF
  - Superficial cervical lnn.: ☐Enlarged Lt., ☐Enlarged Rt., _____ ☐NAF
  - Thyroid:_____ ☐NAF

- Thoracic limb:_____ ☐NAF
  - Foot pads:_____ ☐NAF
  - Knuckling:_____ ☐NAF
  - Axillary lnn. [normally absent]:_____ ☐NAF

- Thorax:_____ ☐NAF

- Abdomen:_____ ☐NAF
  - Mammary chain:_____ ☐NAF
  - Penis/ Testicles/ Vulva:_____ ☐NAF
  - Superficial inguinal lnn. [normally absent]:_____ ☐NAF

- Pelvic limb:_____ ☐NAF
  - Foot pads:_____ ☐NAF
  - Knuckling:_____ ☐NAF
  - Popliteal lnn.: ☐Enlarged Lt., ☐Enlarged Rt., _____ ☐NAF

- Skin:_____ ☐NAF
- Tail:_____ ☐NAF
- Rectal☞⊙:_____ ☐NAF

Problems List:

- **Problem #1**:

- **Problem #2**:

- **Problem #3**:

- **Problem #4**:

- **Problem #5**:

- **Problem #6**:

Diagnostic Plan	Treatment Plan

Case No._____

Patient	Age	Sex		Breed	Weight
		nM	sF		
	DOB:	iM	iF	Color:	kg

Owner	Primary Veterinarian	Admit Date/ Time
Name: Phone:	Name: Phone:	Date: Time: AM / PM

• **Presenting complaint**:_____
_____
_____
_____
_____
_____

• **Medical Hx**:_____
_____
_____
_____
_____
_____

• **When/ where obtained**: Date:_____; ☐Breeder, ☐Shelter, Other:_____

Drug/ Supplement	Amount	Dose (mg/kg)	Route	Frequency	Date Started

• **Vaccine status – Dog**: ☐Rab ☐Parv ☐Dist ☐Aden; ☐Para ☐Lep ☐Bord ☐Influ ☐Lyme
• **Vaccine status – Cat**: ☐Rab ☐Herp ☐Cali ☐Pan ☐FeLV [kittens]; ☐FIV ☐Chlam ☐Bord
• **Heartworm / Flea & Tick / Intestinal Parasites**:
  ◦ *Last Heartworm Test*: Date:_____, ☐IDK; Test Results: ☐Pos, ☐Neg, ☐IDK
  ◦ *Monthly heartworm preventative*: ☐no ☐yes, Product:_____
  ◦ *Monthly flea & tick preventative*: ☐no ☐yes, Product:_____
  ◦ *Monthly dewormer*:   ☐no ☐yes, Product:_____
• **Surgical Hx**: ☐Spay/Neuter; Date:_____; Other:_____
• **Environment**: ☐Indoor, ☐Outdoor, Time spent outdoors/ Other:_____
• **Housemates**: Dogs:_____ Cats:_____ Other:_____
• **Diet**: ☐Wet, ☐Dry; Brand/ Amt.:_____

Appetite	☐Normal, ☐↑, ☐↓
Weight	☐Normal, ☐↑, ☐↓; Past Wt.:_____ kg; Date:_____; Δ:_____
Thirst	☐Normal, ☐↑, ☐↓
Urination	☐Normal, ☐↑, ☐↓, ☐Blood, ☐Strain
Defecation	☐Normal, ☐↑, ☐↓, ☐Blood, ☐Strain, ☐Diarrhea, ☐Mucus
Discharge	☐No, ☐Yes; Onset/ Describe:
Cough/ Sneeze	☐No, ☐Yes; Onset/ Describe:
Vomit	☐No, ☐Yes; Onset/ Describe:
Respiration	☐Normal, ☐↑ Rate, ☐↑ Effort
Energy level	☐Normal, ☐Lethargic, ☐Exercise intolerance

• **Travel Hx**: ☐None, Other:_____
• **Exposure to**: ☐Standing water, ☐Wildlife, ☐Board/daycare, ☐Dog park, ☐Groomer, ☐Pet store
• **Adverse reactions to food/ meds**: ☐None, Other:_____
• **Can give oral meds**: ☐no ☐yes; Helpful Tricks:_____

Physical Exam – General:

- **Body Weight:**_____kg   **Body Condition Score:**___/9

- **Temperature:**_____°F [*Dog-RI*: 100.9–102.4; *Cat-RI*: 98.1–102.1]

- **Heart:**
  - *Rate*:_____beats/min [Dog-RI: 60–180; Cat-RI: 140–240 (in hospital)]
  - *Rhythm*: ☐Regular, ☐Irregular
  - *Sounds*: ☐None, ☐Split sound[S1 or S2], ☐Gallop[S3 or S4], ☐Murmur, ☐Muffled
    - *Grade*: ☐1–2[soft, only at PMI], ☐3–4[moderate, mild radiate], ☐5–6[loud, strong radiate, thrill]
    - *Timing*: ☐Systolic, ☐Diastolic, ☐Continuous
    - *PMI*:

	PMI	Over	Anatomic Boundaries
☐	Lt. apex	Mitral valve	5th to 6th ICS at level of CCJ
☐	Lt. base	Ao + Pul outflow	2nd to 4th ICS above the CCJ
☐	Rt. midheart	Tricuspid valve	3rd to 5th ICS near the CCJ
☐	Rt. sternal border	Right ventricle	5th to 7th ICS immediately dorsal to the sternum
☐	Sternal (cat)	Sternum	In cats, determination of PMI offers very little clinical significance.

  - *Vertebral Heart Size*: Dog = 8.7–10.7; Cat = 6.9–8.1 (from cranial edge of T4)
  - *Innocent Murmur*: Grade 1-2, systolic, left base location, disappear by ~4 months of age, absent clinical signs

- **Pulses:**
  - *Pulse rate*:_____pulses/min
  - *Character*: ☐Sync, ☐Async; ☐Normokinetic, ☐Hyper-, ☐Hypo-, ☐Variable

- **Lungs:**
  - *Respiratory rate*:_____breaths/min [RI: 16–30]
  - *Depth/Effort*: ☐Norm, ☐Pant, ☐Deep, ☐Shallow, ☐↑ Insp. effort, ☐↑ Exp. effort
  - *Sounds/Localization*:
    - ☐Norm BV, ☐Quiet BV, ☐Loud BV, ☐Crack, ☐Wheez, ☐Frict, ☐Muffled
    - ☐All lung fields, ☐Rt cran, ☐Rt mid, ☐Rt caud, ☐Lt cran, ☐Lt mid, ☐Lt caud
  - *Tracheal Auscultation/ Palpation*: ☐Normal, Other:_____

- **Pain Score:**_____ / 5   Localization:_____

- **Mentation:** ☐BAR ☐Confused/ ☐Drowsy/ ☐Stuporous ☐Coma
  - ☐QAR   Disoriented   Obtunded   (unresponsive unless   (complete
  - ☐Dull   (conscious; inappropriate   (↓ interaction with   aroused by noxious   unresponsiveness
  - (conscious; responds   response to environment   environment; slow   stimuli)   to any stimuli)
  - to sensory stimuli)   [ex., vocalization, head   response to verbal
  -    pressing])   stimuli)

- **Skin Elasticity:** ☐Normal skin turgor, ☐↓ Skin turgor, ☐Skin tent, ☐Gelatinous

- **Mucus Membranes:**
  - *CRT*:_____ [RI: 1–2; <1 = compensated shock, sepsis, heat stroke; <2 = acute decompensated shock; >2 = late decompensated shock, decreased cardiac output, hypothermia]
  - *Color*:_____ [RI: pink; red = compensated shock, sepsis, heat stroke; pale/white = anemia, shock; blue = cyanosis; yellow = hepatic disease, extravascular hemolysis; brown = met-Hb]
  - *Texture*:_____ [RI: moist = hydrated; tacky-to-dry = 5–12% dehydrated]

Physical Exam – Systems Checklist:

- **Head:**_____ ☐NAF
  - ○ Ears: ☐Ceruminous debris (mild / mod / sev) (AS / AD / AU), _____ ☐NAF
  - ○ Eyes:_____ ☐NAF
    - ▪ Retinal:_____ ☐NAF

→ Ⓛ		Ⓡ		Ⓛ		Ⓡ ←	
☐ ⊙ Normal Direct	☐ ⊙ Normal Indirect	☐ ⊙ Normal Indirect	☐ ⊙ Normal Direct
☐ ⦿ Abnormal Direct	☐ ⦿ Abnormal Indirect	☐ ⦿ Abnormal Indirect	☐ ⦿ Abnormal Direct

  - ○ Nose:_____ ☐NAF
  - ○ Oral cavity: ☐Tarter/Gingivitis (mild / mod / sev), _____ ☐NAF
  - ○ Mandibular lnn.: ☐Enlarged Lt., ☐Enlarged Rt., _____ ☐NAF

- **Neck:**_____ ☐NAF
  - ○ Superficial cervical lnn.: ☐Enlarged Lt., ☐Enlarged Rt., _____ ☐NAF
  - ○ Thyroid:_____ ☐NAF

- **Thoracic limb:**_____ ☐NAF
  - ○ Foot pads:_____ ☐NAF
  - ○ Knuckling:_____ ☐NAF
  - ○ Axillary lnn. [normally absent]:_____ ☐NAF

- **Thorax:**_____ ☐NAF

- **Abdomen:**_____ ☐NAF
  - ○ Mammary chain:_____ ☐NAF
  - ○ Penis/ Testicles/ Vulva:_____ ☐NAF
  - ○ Superficial inguinal lnn. [normally absent]:_____ ☐NAF

- **Pelvic limb:**_____ ☐NAF
  - ○ Foot pads:_____ ☐NAF
  - ○ Knuckling:_____ ☐NAF
  - ○ Popliteal lnn.: ☐Enlarged Lt., ☐Enlarged Rt., _____ ☐NAF

- **Skin:**_____ ☐NAF
- **Tail:**_____ ☐NAF
- **Rectal☞⊙:**_____ ☐NAF

Problems List:

- **Problem #1:**

- **Problem #2:**

- **Problem #3:**

- **Problem #4:**

- **Problem #5:**

- **Problem #6:**

Diagnostic Plan	Treatment Plan

Case No._____

Patient	Age	Sex		Breed		Weight
		nM	sF			
	DOB:	iM	iF	Color:		kg

Owner		Primary Veterinarian		Admit Date/ Time	
Name:		Name:		Date:	
Phone:		Phone:		Time:	AM / PM

- **Presenting complaint**:_____
_____
_____
_____
_____
_____

- **Medical Hx**:_____
_____
_____
_____
_____

- **When/ where obtained**: Date:_____ ; ☐Breeder, ☐Shelter, Other:_____

Drug/ Supplement	Amount	Dose (mg/kg)	Route	Frequency	Date Started

- **Vaccine status – Dog**: ☐Rab ☐Parv ☐Dist ☐Aden; ☐Para ☐Lep ☐Bord ☐Influ ☐Lyme
- **Vaccine status – Cat**: ☐Rab ☐Herp ☐Cali ☐Pan ☐FeLV [kittens]; ☐FIV ☐Chlam ☐Bord
- **Heartworm / Flea & Tick / Intestinal Parasites**:
  - *Last Heartworm Test*: Date:_____, ☐IDK; Test Results: ☐Pos, ☐Neg, ☐IDK
  - *Monthly heartworm preventative*: ☐no ☐yes, Product:_____
  - *Monthly flea & tick preventative*: ☐no ☐yes, Product:_____
  - *Monthly dewormer*: ☐no ☐yes, Product:_____
- **Surgical Hx**: ☐Spay/Neuter; Date:_____; Other:_____
- **Environment**: ☐Indoor, ☐Outdoor, Time spent outdoors/ Other:_____
- **Housemates**: Dogs:_____ Cats:_____ Other:_____
- **Diet**: ☐Wet, ☐Dry; Brand/ Amt.:_____

Appetite	☐Normal, ☐↑, ☐↓
Weight	☐Normal, ☐↑, ☐↓; Past Wt.:_____ kg; Date:_____; Δ:_____
Thirst	☐Normal, ☐↑, ☐↓
Urination	☐Normal, ☐↑, ☐↓, ☐Blood, ☐Strain
Defecation	☐Normal, ☐↑, ☐↓, ☐Blood, ☐Strain, ☐Diarrhea, ☐Mucus
Discharge	☐No, ☐Yes; Onset/ Describe:
Cough/ Sneeze	☐No, ☐Yes; Onset/ Describe:
Vomit	☐No, ☐Yes; Onset/ Describe:
Respiration	☐Normal, ☐↑ Rate, ☐↑ Effort
Energy level	☐Normal, ☐Lethargic, ☐Exercise intolerance

- **Travel Hx**: ☐None, Other:_____
- **Exposure to**: ☐Standing water, ☐Wildlife, ☐Board/daycare, ☐Dog park, ☐Groomer, ☐Pet store
- **Adverse reactions to food/ meds**: ☐None, Other:_____
- **Can give oral meds**: ☐no ☐yes; Helpful Tricks:_____

Physical Exam – General:

- **Body Weight**:_____kg   **Body Condition Score**:___/9

- **Temperature**:_____°F [*Dog-RI*: 100.9–102.4;   *Cat-RI*: 98.1–102.1]

- **Heart**:
  - *Rate*:_____beats/min [Dog-RI: 60–180;   Cat-RI: 140–240 (in hospital)]
  - *Rhythm*: ☐Regular, ☐Irregular
  - *Sounds*: ☐None, ☐Split sound[S1 or S2], ☐Gallop[S3 or S4], ☐Murmur, ☐Muffled
    - *Grade*: ☐1–2[soft, only at PMI],   ☐3–4[moderate, mild radiate],   ☐5–6[loud, strong radiate, thrill]
    - *Timing*: ☐Systolic, ☐Diastolic, ☐Continuous
    - *PMI*:

	PMI	Over	Anatomic Boundaries
☐	Lt. apex	Mitral valve	5th to 6th ICS at level of CCJ
☐	Lt. base	Ao + Pul outflow	2nd to 4th ICS above the CCJ
☐	Rt. midheart	Tricuspid valve	3rd to 5th ICS near the CCJ
☐	Rt. sternal border	Right ventricle	5th to 7th ICS immediately dorsal to the sternum
☐	Sternal (cat)	Sternum	In cats, determination of PMI offers very little clinical significance.

-      •   *Vertebral Heart Size*: Dog = 8.7–10.7; Cat = 6.9–8.1 (from cranial edge of T4)
-      •   *Innocent Murmur*: Grade 1-2, systolic, left base location, disappear by ~4 months of age, absent clinical signs

- **Pulses**:
  - *Pulse rate*:_____pulses/min
  - *Character*: ☐Sync, ☐Async;   ☐Normokinetic, ☐Hyper-, ☐Hypo-, ☐Variable

- **Lungs**:
  - *Respiratory rate*:_____breaths/min [*RI*: 16–30]
  - *Depth/Effort*: ☐Norm, ☐Pant, ☐Deep, ☐Shallow, ☐↑ Insp. effort, ☐↑ Exp. effort
  - *Sounds/Localization*:
    - ☐Norm BV, ☐Quiet BV, ☐Loud BV, ☐Crack, ☐Wheez, ☐Frict, ☐Muffled
    - ☐All lung fields, ☐Rt cran, ☐Rt mid, ☐Rt caud, ☐Lt cran, ☐Lt mid, ☐Lt caud
  - *Tracheal Auscultation/ Palpation*: ☐Normal, Other:_____

- **Pain Score**:_____ / 5   Localization:_____

- **Mentation**:

☐BAR	☐Confused/	☐Drowsy/	☐Stuporous	☐Coma
☐QAR	Disoriented	Obtunded	(unresponsive unless	(complete
☐Dull	(conscious; inappropriate	(↓ interaction with	aroused by noxious	unresponsiveness
(conscious; responds	response to environment	environment; slow	stimuli)	to any stimuli)
to sensory stimuli)	[ex., vocalization, head	response to verbal		
	pressing])	stimuli)		

- **Skin Elasticity**: ☐Normal skin turgor, ☐↓ Skin turgor, ☐Skin tent, ☐Gelatinous

- **Mucus Membranes**:
  - *CRT*:_____ [*RI*: 1–2; <1 = compensated shock, sepsis, heat stroke; <2 = acute decompensated shock; >2 = late decompensated shock, decreased cardiac output, hypothermia]
  - *Color*:_____ [*RI*: pink; red = compensated shock, sepsis, heat stroke; pale/white = anemia, shock; blue = cyanosis; yellow = hepatic disease, extravascular hemolysis; brown = met-Hb]
  - *Texture*:_____ [*RI*: moist = hydrated; tacky-to-dry = 5–12% dehydrated]

Physical Exam – Systems Checklist:

• Head:_____ ☐NAF
  ◦ Ears: ☐Ceruminous debris (mild / mod / sev) (AS / AD / AU), _____ ☐NAF
  ◦ Eyes:_____ ☐NAF
    ▪ Retinal:_____ ☐NAF

→ Ⓛ		Ⓡ		Ⓛ		Ⓡ ←	
☐	◉ Normal Direct	☐	◉ Normal Indirect	☐	◉ Normal Indirect	☐	◉ Normal Direct
☐	◉ Abnormal Direct	☐	◉ Abnormal Indirect	☐	◉ Abnormal Indirect	☐	◉ Abnormal Direct

  ◦ Nose:_____ ☐NAF
  ◦ Oral cavity: ☐Tarter/Gingivitis (mild / mod / sev), _____ ☐NAF
  ◦ Mandibular lnn.: ☐Enlarged Lt., ☐Enlarged Rt., _____ ☐NAF

• Neck:_____ ☐NAF
  ◦ Superficial cervical lnn.: ☐Enlarged Lt., ☐Enlarged Rt., _____ ☐NAF
  ◦ Thyroid:_____ ☐NAF

• Thoracic limb:_____ ☐NAF
  ◦ Foot pads:_____ ☐NAF
  ◦ Knuckling:_____ ☐NAF
  ◦ Axillary lnn. [normally absent]:_____ ☐NAF

• Thorax:_____ ☐NAF

• Abdomen:_____ ☐NAF
  ◦ Mammary chain:_____ ☐NAF
  ◦ Penis/ Testicles/ Vulva:_____ ☐NAF
  ◦ Superficial inguinal lnn. [normally absent]:_____ ☐NAF

• Pelvic limb:_____ ☐NAF
  ◦ Foot pads:_____ ☐NAF
  ◦ Knuckling:_____ ☐NAF
  ◦ Popliteal lnn.: ☐Enlarged Lt., ☐Enlarged Rt., _____ ☐NAF

• Skin:_____ ☐NAF
• Tail:_____ ☐NAF
• Rectal☞⊙:_____ ☐NAF

Problems List:

- **Problem #1**:

- **Problem #2**:

- **Problem #3**:

- **Problem #4**:

- **Problem #5**:

- **Problem #6**:

Diagnostic Plan	Treatment Plan

Case No._____

Patient	Age	Sex		Breed	Weight
		nM	sF		
	DOB:	iM	iF	Color:	kg

Owner	Primary Veterinarian	Admit Date/ Time
Name: Phone:	Name: Phone:	Date: Time: AM / PM

• **Presenting complaint**:_____
_____
_____
_____
_____

• **Medical Hx**:_____
_____
_____
_____
_____

• **When/ where obtained**: Date:_____; ☐Breeder, ☐Shelter, Other:_____

Drug/ Supplement	Amount	Dose (mg/kg)	Route	Frequency	Date Started

• **Vaccine status – Dog**: ☐Rab ☐Parv ☐Dist ☐Aden; ☐Para ☐Lep ☐Bord ☐Influ ☐Lyme
• **Vaccine status – Cat**: ☐Rab ☐Herp ☐Cali ☐Pan ☐FeLV [kittens]; ☐FIV ☐Chlam ☐Bord
• **Heartworm / Flea & Tick / Intestinal Parasites**:
  ◦ *Last Heartworm Test*: Date:_____, ☐IDK; Test Results: ☐Pos, ☐Neg, ☐IDK
  ◦ *Monthly heartworm preventative*: ☐no ☐yes, Product:_____
  ◦ *Monthly flea & tick preventative*: ☐no ☐yes, Product:_____
  ◦ *Monthly dewormer*:   ☐no ☐yes, Product:_____
• **Surgical Hx**: ☐Spay/Neuter; Date:_____; Other:_____
• **Environment**: ☐Indoor, ☐Outdoor, Time spent outdoors/ Other:_____
• **Housemates**: Dogs:_____ Cats:_____ Other:_____
• **Diet**: ☐Wet, ☐Dry; Brand/ Amt.:_____

Appetite	☐Normal, ☐↑, ☐↓
Weight	☐Normal, ☐↑, ☐↓; Past Wt.:_____ kg; Date:_____; Δ:_____
Thirst	☐Normal, ☐↑, ☐↓
Urination	☐Normal, ☐↑, ☐↓, ☐Blood, ☐Strain
Defecation	☐Normal, ☐↑, ☐↓, ☐Blood, ☐Strain, ☐Diarrhea, ☐Mucus
Discharge	☐No, ☐Yes; Onset/ Describe:
Cough/ Sneeze	☐No, ☐Yes; Onset/ Describe:
Vomit	☐No, ☐Yes; Onset/ Describe:
Respiration	☐Normal, ☐↑ Rate, ☐↑ Effort
Energy level	☐Normal, ☐Lethargic, ☐Exercise intolerance

• **Travel Hx**: ☐None, Other:_____
• **Exposure to**: ☐Standing water, ☐Wildlife, ☐Board/daycare, ☐Dog park, ☐Groomer, ☐Pet store
• **Adverse reactions to food/ meds**: ☐None, Other:_____
• **Can give oral meds**: ☐no ☐yes; Helpful Tricks:_____

Physical Exam – General:

- **Body Weight**:_____kg   **Body Condition Score**:___/9

- **Temperature**:_____°F [*Dog-RI*: 100.9–102.4; *Cat-RI*: 98.1–102.1]

- **Heart**:
  - *Rate*:_____beats/min [Dog-RI: 60–180; Cat-RI: 140–240 (in hospital)]
  - *Rhythm*: □Regular, □Irregular
  - *Sounds*: □None, □Split sound[S1 or S2], □Gallop[S3 or S4], □Murmur, □Muffled
    - *Grade*: □1–2[soft, only at PMI],   □3–4[moderate, mild radiate],   □5–6[loud, strong radiate, thrill]
    - *Timing*: □Systolic, □Diastolic, □Continuous
    - *PMI*:

	PMI	Over	Anatomic Boundaries
□	Lt. apex	Mitral valve	5th to 6th ICS at level of CCJ
□	Lt. base	Ao + Pul outflow	2nd to 4th ICS above the CCJ
□	Rt. midheart	Tricuspid valve	3rd to 5th ICS near the CCJ
□	Rt. sternal border	Right ventricle	5th to 7th ICS immediately dorsal to the sternum
□	Sternal (cat)	Sternum	In cats, determination of PMI offers very little clinical significance.

  - • *Vertebral Heart Size*: Dog = 8.7–10.7; Cat = 6.9–8.1 (from cranial edge of T4)
  - • *Innocent Murmur*: Grade 1-2, systolic, left base location, disappear by ~4 months of age, absent clinical signs

- **Pulses**:
  - *Pulse rate*:_____pulses/min
  - *Character*: □Sync, □Async; □Normokinetic, □Hyper-, □Hypo-, □Variable

- **Lungs**:
  - *Respiratory rate*:_____breaths/min [*RI*: 16–30]
  - *Depth/Effort*: □Norm, □Pant, □Deep, □Shallow, □↑ Insp. effort, □↑ Exp. effort
  - *Sounds/Localization*:
    - □Norm BV, □Quiet BV, □Loud BV, □Crack, □Wheez, □Frict, □Muffled
    - □All lung fields, □Rt cran, □Rt mid, □Rt caud, □Lt cran, □Lt mid, □Lt caud
  - *Tracheal Auscultation/ Palpation*: □Normal, Other:_____

- **Pain Score**:_____ / 5   Localization:_____

- **Mentation**: □BAR   □Confused/   □Drowsy/   □Stuporous   □Coma
  □QAR   Disoriented   Obtunded   (unresponsive unless   (complete
  □Dull   (conscious; inappropriate   (↓ interaction with   aroused by noxious   unresponsiveness
  (conscious; responds   response to environment   environment; slow   stimuli)   to any stimuli)
  to sensory stimuli)   [ex., vocalization, head   response to verbal
                        pressing])   stimuli)

- **Skin Elasticity**: □Normal skin turgor, □↓ Skin turgor, □Skin tent, □Gelatinous

- **Mucus Membranes**:
  - *CRT*:_____ [*RI*: 1–2; <1 = compensated shock, sepsis, heat stroke; <2 = acute decompensated shock; >2 = late decompensated shock, decreased cardiac output, hypothermia]
  - *Color*:_____ [*RI*: pink; red = compensated shock, sepsis, heat stroke; pale/white = anemia, shock; blue = cyanosis; yellow = hepatic disease, extravascular hemolysis; brown = met-Hb]
  - *Texture*:_____ [*RI*: moist = hydrated; tacky-to-dry = 5–12% dehydrated]

Physical Exam – Systems Checklist:

• Head:_____ □NAF
    ◦ Ears: □Ceruminous debris (mild / mod / sev) (AS / AD / AU), _____ □NAF
    ◦ Eyes:_____ □NAF
       ▪ Retinal:_____ □NAF

→ Ⓛ		Ⓡ		Ⓛ		Ⓡ ←	
□ ⊙ Normal Direct	□ ⊙ Normal Indirect	□ ⊙ Normal Indirect	□ ⊙ Normal Direct
□ ⊙ Abnormal Direct	□ ⊙ Abnormal Indirect	□ ⊙ Abnormal Indirect	□ ⊙ Abnormal Direct

    ◦ Nose:_____ □NAF
    ◦ Oral cavity: □Tarter/Gingivitis (mild / mod / sev), _____ □NAF
    ◦ Mandibular lnn.: □Enlarged Lt., □Enlarged Rt., _____ □NAF

• Neck:_____ □NAF
    ◦ Superficial cervical lnn.: □Enlarged Lt., □Enlarged Rt., _____ □NAF
    ◦ Thyroid:_____ □NAF

• Thoracic limb:_____ □NAF
    ◦ Foot pads:_____ □NAF
    ◦ Knuckling:_____ □NAF
    ◦ Axillary lnn. [normally absent]:_____ □NAF

• Thorax:_____ □NAF

• Abdomen:_____ □NAF
    ◦ Mammary chain:_____ □NAF
    ◦ Penis/ Testicles/ Vulva:_____ □NAF
    ◦ Superficial inguinal lnn. [normally absent]:_____ □NAF

• Pelvic limb:_____ □NAF
    ◦ Foot pads:_____ □NAF
    ◦ Knuckling:_____ □NAF
    ◦ Popliteal lnn.: □Enlarged Lt., □Enlarged Rt., _____ □NAF

• Skin:_____ □NAF
• Tail:_____ □NAF
• Rectal☞⊙:_____ □NAF

Problems List:

- **Problem #1**:

- **Problem #2**:

- **Problem #3**:

- **Problem #4**:

- **Problem #5**:

- **Problem #6**:

Diagnostic Plan	Treatment Plan

Case No._____

Patient	Age	Sex		Breed	Weight
		nM	sF		
	DOB:	iM	iF	Color:	kg

Owner	Primary Veterinarian	Admit Date/ Time
Name: Phone:	Name: Phone:	Date: Time: AM / PM

• **Presenting complaint**:_____
_____
_____
_____
_____
_____

• **Medical Hx**:_____
_____
_____
_____
_____
_____

• **When/ where obtained**: Date:_____; ☐Breeder, ☐Shelter, Other:_____

Drug/ Supplement	Amount	Dose (mg/kg)	Route	Frequency	Date Started

• **Vaccine status – Dog**: ☐Rab ☐Parv ☐Dist ☐Aden; ☐Para ☐Lep ☐Bord ☐Influ ☐Lyme
• **Vaccine status – Cat**: ☐Rab ☐Herp ☐Cali ☐Pan ☐FeLV [kittens]; ☐FIV ☐Chlam ☐Bord
• **Heartworm / Flea & Tick / Intestinal Parasites**:
  ◦ *Last Heartworm Test*: Date:_____, ☐IDK; Test Results: ☐Pos, ☐Neg, ☐IDK
  ◦ *Monthly heartworm preventative*: ☐no ☐yes, Product:_____
  ◦ *Monthly flea & tick preventative*: ☐no ☐yes, Product:_____
  ◦ *Monthly dewormer*:   ☐no ☐yes, Product:_____
• **Surgical Hx**: ☐Spay/Neuter; Date:_____; Other:_____
• **Environment**: ☐Indoor, ☐Outdoor, Time spent outdoors/ Other:_____
• **Housemates**: Dogs:_____ Cats:_____ Other:_____
• **Diet**: ☐Wet, ☐Dry; Brand/ Amt.:_____

Appetite	☐Normal, ☐↑, ☐↓
Weight	☐Normal, ☐↑, ☐↓; Past Wt.:_____ kg; Date:_____; Δ:_____
Thirst	☐Normal, ☐↑, ☐↓
Urination	☐Normal, ☐↑, ☐↓, ☐Blood, ☐Strain
Defecation	☐Normal, ☐↑, ☐↓, ☐Blood, ☐Strain, ☐Diarrhea, ☐Mucus
Discharge	☐No, ☐Yes; Onset/ Describe:
Cough/ Sneeze	☐No, ☐Yes; Onset/ Describe:
Vomit	☐No, ☐Yes; Onset/ Describe:
Respiration	☐Normal, ☐↑ Rate, ☐↑ Effort
Energy level	☐Normal, ☐Lethargic, ☐Exercise intolerance

• **Travel Hx**: ☐None, Other:_____
• **Exposure to**: ☐Standing water, ☐Wildlife, ☐Board/daycare, ☐Dog park, ☐Groomer, ☐Pet store
• **Adverse reactions to food/ meds**: ☐None, Other:_____
• **Can give oral meds**: ☐no ☐yes; Helpful Tricks:_____

Physical Exam – General:

- **Body Weight**:_____kg   **Body Condition Score**:___/9

- **Temperature**:_____°F [*Dog-RI*: 100.9–102.4; *Cat-RI*: 98.1–102.1]

- **Heart**:
  - *Rate*:_____beats/min [Dog-RI: 60–180; Cat-RI: 140–240 (in hospital)]
  - *Rhythm*: ☐Regular, ☐Irregular
  - *Sounds*: ☐None, ☐Split sound[S1 or S2], ☐Gallop[S3 or S4], ☐Murmur, ☐Muffled
    - *Grade*: ☐1–2[soft, only at PMI],   ☐3–4[moderate, mild radiate],   ☐5–6[loud, strong radiate, thrill]
    - *Timing*: ☐Systolic, ☐Diastolic, ☐Continuous
    - *PMI*:

	PMI	Over	Anatomic Boundaries
☐	Lt. apex	Mitral valve	5th to 6th ICS at level of CCJ
☐	Lt. base	Ao + Pul outflow	2nd to 4th ICS above the CCJ
☐	Rt. midheart	Tricuspid valve	3rd to 5th ICS near the CCJ
☐	Rt. sternal border	Right ventricle	5th to 7th ICS immediately dorsal to the sternum
☐	Sternal (cat)	Sternum	In cats, determination of PMI offers very little clinical significance.

  - *Vertebral Heart Size*: Dog = 8.7–10.7; Cat = 6.9–8.1 (from cranial edge of T4)
  - *Innocent Murmur*: Grade 1-2, systolic, left base location, disappear by ~4 months of age, absent clinical signs

- **Pulses**:
  - *Pulse rate*:_____pulses/min
  - *Character*: ☐Sync, ☐Async; ☐Normokinetic, ☐Hyper-, ☐Hypo-, ☐Variable

- **Lungs**:
  - *Respiratory rate*:_____breaths/min [*RI*: 16–30]
  - *Depth/Effort*: ☐Norm, ☐Pant, ☐Deep, ☐Shallow, ☐↑ Insp. effort, ☐↑ Exp. effort
  - *Sounds/Localization*:
    - ☐Norm BV, ☐Quiet BV, ☐Loud BV, ☐Crack, ☐Wheez, ☐Frict, ☐Muffled
    - ☐All lung fields, ☐Rt cran, ☐Rt mid, ☐Rt caud, ☐Lt cran, ☐Lt mid, ☐Lt caud
  - *Tracheal Auscultation/ Palpation*: ☐Normal, Other:_____

- **Pain Score**:_____ / 5   Localization:_____

- **Mentation**:

☐BAR ☐QAR ☐Dull (conscious; responds to sensory stimuli)	☐Confused/ Disoriented (conscious; inappropriate response to environment [ex., vocalization, head pressing])	☐Drowsy/ Obtunded (↓ interaction with environment; slow response to verbal stimuli)	☐Stuporous (unresponsive unless aroused by noxious stimuli)	☐Coma (complete unresponsiveness to any stimuli)

- **Skin Elasticity**: ☐Normal skin turgor, ☐↓ Skin turgor, ☐Skin tent, ☐Gelatinous

- **Mucus Membranes**:
  - *CRT*:_____ [*RI*: 1–2; <1 = compensated shock, sepsis, heat stroke; <2 = acute decompensated shock; >2 = late decompensated shock, decreased cardiac output, hypothermia]
  - *Color*:_____ [*RI*: pink; red = compensated shock, sepsis, heat stroke; pale/white = anemia, shock; blue = cyanosis; yellow = hepatic disease, extravascular hemolysis; brown = met-Hb]
  - *Texture*:_____ [*RI*: moist = hydrated; tacky-to-dry = 5–12% dehydrated]

Physical Exam – Systems Checklist:

- Head: _____ ☐NAF
  - ◦ Ears: ☐Ceruminous debris (mild / mod / sev) (AS / AD / AU), _____ ☐NAF
  - ◦ Eyes: _____ ☐NAF
    - ▪ Retinal: _____ ☐NAF

→Ⓛ		Ⓡ		Ⓛ		Ⓡ←	
☐	Normal Direct	☐	Normal Indirect	☐	Normal Indirect	☐	Normal Direct
☐	Abnormal Direct	☐	Abnormal Indirect	☐	Abnormal Indirect	☐	Abnormal Direct

  - ◦ Nose: _____ ☐NAF
  - ◦ Oral cavity: ☐Tarter/Gingivitis (mild / mod / sev), _____ ☐NAF
  - ◦ Mandibular lnn.: ☐Enlarged Lt., ☐Enlarged Rt., _____ ☐NAF

- Neck: _____ ☐NAF
  - ◦ Superficial cervical lnn.: ☐Enlarged Lt., ☐Enlarged Rt., _____ ☐NAF
  - ◦ Thyroid: _____ ☐NAF

- Thoracic limb: _____ ☐NAF
  - ◦ Foot pads: _____ ☐NAF
  - ◦ Knuckling: _____ ☐NAF
  - ◦ Axillary lnn. [normally absent]: _____ ☐NAF

- Thorax: _____ ☐NAF

- Abdomen: _____ ☐NAF
  - ◦ Mammary chain: _____ ☐NAF
  - ◦ Penis/ Testicles/ Vulva: _____ ☐NAF
  - ◦ Superficial inguinal lnn. [normally absent]: _____ ☐NAF

- Pelvic limb: _____ ☐NAF
  - ◦ Foot pads: _____ ☐NAF
  - ◦ Knuckling: _____ ☐NAF
  - ◦ Popliteal lnn.: ☐Enlarged Lt., ☐Enlarged Rt., _____ ☐NAF

- Skin: _____ ☐NAF
- Tail: _____ ☐NAF
- Rectal☞☉: _____ ☐NAF

Problems List:

- **Problem #1**:

- **Problem #2**:

- **Problem #3**:

- **Problem #4**:

- **Problem #5**:

- **Problem #6**:

Diagnostic Plan	Treatment Plan

Case No._____

Patient	Age	Sex		Breed	Weight
		nM	sF		
	DOB:	iM	iF	Color:	kg

Owner	Primary Veterinarian	Admit Date/ Time
Name: Phone:	Name: Phone:	Date: Time: AM / PM

• Presenting complaint:_____
_____
_____
_____
_____
_____

• Medical Hx:_____
_____
_____
_____
_____

• When/ where obtained: Date:_____; ☐Breeder, ☐Shelter, Other:_____

Drug/ Supplement	Amount	Dose (mg/kg)	Route	Frequency	Date Started

• Vaccine status – Dog: ☐Rab ☐Parv ☐Dist ☐Aden; ☐Para ☐Lep ☐Bord ☐Influ ☐Lyme
• Vaccine status – Cat: ☐Rab ☐Herp ☐Cali ☐Pan ☐FeLV [kittens]; ☐FIV ☐Chlam ☐Bord
• Heartworm / Flea & Tick / Intestinal Parasites:
   ◦ *Last Heartworm Test*: Date:_____, ☐IDK; Test Results: ☐Pos, ☐Neg, ☐IDK
   ◦ *Monthly heartworm preventative*: ☐no ☐yes, Product:_____
   ◦ *Monthly flea & tick preventative*: ☐no ☐yes, Product:_____
   ◦ *Monthly dewormer*: ☐no ☐yes, Product:_____
• Surgical Hx: ☐Spay/Neuter; Date:_____; Other:_____
• Environment: ☐Indoor, ☐Outdoor, Time spent outdoors/ Other:_____
• Housemates: Dogs:_____ Cats:_____ Other:_____
• Diet: ☐Wet, ☐Dry; Brand/ Amt.:_____

Appetite	☐Normal, ☐↑, ☐↓
Weight	☐Normal, ☐↑, ☐↓; Past Wt.:_____ kg; Date:_____; Δ:_____
Thirst	☐Normal, ☐↑, ☐↓
Urination	☐Normal, ☐↑, ☐↓, ☐Blood, ☐Strain
Defecation	☐Normal, ☐↑, ☐↓, ☐Blood, ☐Strain, ☐Diarrhea, ☐Mucus
Discharge	☐No, ☐Yes; Onset/ Describe:
Cough/ Sneeze	☐No, ☐Yes; Onset/ Describe:
Vomit	☐No, ☐Yes; Onset/ Describe:
Respiration	☐Normal, ☐↑ Rate, ☐↑ Effort
Energy level	☐Normal, ☐Lethargic, ☐Exercise intolerance

• Travel Hx: ☐None, Other:_____
• Exposure to: ☐Standing water, ☐Wildlife, ☐Board/daycare, ☐Dog park, ☐Groomer, ☐Pet store
• Adverse reactions to food/ meds: ☐None, Other:_____
• Can give oral meds: ☐no ☐yes; Helpful Tricks:_____

Physical Exam – General:

- **Body Weight**:_____kg **Body Condition Score**:___/9

- **Temperature**:_____°F [*Dog-RI*: 100.9–102.4; *Cat-RI*: 98.1–102.1]

- **Heart**:
  - *Rate*:_____beats/min [Dog-RI: 60–180; Cat-RI: 140–240 (in hospital)]
  - *Rhythm*: ☐Regular, ☐Irregular
  - *Sounds*: ☐None, ☐Split sound[S1 or S2], ☐Gallop[S3 or S4], ☐Murmur, ☐Muffled
    - *Grade*: ☐1–2[soft, only at PMI],   ☐3–4[moderate, mild radiate],   ☐5–6[loud, strong radiate, thrill]
    - *Timing*: ☐Systolic, ☐Diastolic, ☐Continuous
    - *PMI*:

	PMI	Over	Anatomic Boundaries
☐	Lt. apex	Mitral valve	5th to 6th ICS at level of CCJ
☐	Lt. base	Ao + Pul outflow	2nd to 4th ICS above the CCJ
☐	Rt. midheart	Tricuspid valve	3rd to 5th ICS near the CCJ
☐	Rt. sternal border	Right ventricle	5th to 7th ICS immediately dorsal to the sternum
☐	Sternal (cat)	Sternum	In cats, determination of PMI offers very little clinical significance.

  - *Vertebral Heart Size*: Dog = 8.7–10.7; Cat = 6.9–8.1 (from cranial edge of T4)
  - *Innocent Murmur*: Grade 1-2, systolic, left base location, disappear by ~4 months of age, absent clinical signs

- **Pulses**:
  - *Pulse rate*:_____pulses/min
  - *Character*: ☐Sync, ☐Async; ☐Normokinetic, ☐Hyper-, ☐Hypo-, ☐Variable

- **Lungs**:
  - *Respiratory rate*:_____breaths/min [*RI*: 16–30]
  - *Depth/Effort*: ☐Norm, ☐Pant, ☐Deep, ☐Shallow, ☐↑ Insp. effort, ☐↑ Exp. effort
  - *Sounds/Localization*:
    - ☐Norm BV, ☐Quiet BV, ☐Loud BV, ☐Crack, ☐Wheez, ☐Frict, ☐Muffled
    - ☐All lung fields, ☐Rt cran, ☐Rt mid, ☐Rt caud, ☐Lt cran, ☐Lt mid, ☐Lt caud
  - *Tracheal Auscultation/ Palpation*: ☐Normal, Other:_____

- **Pain Score**:_____ / 5   Localization:_____

- **Mentation**:

☐BAR ☐QAR ☐Dull (conscious; responds to sensory stimuli)	☐Confused/ Disoriented (conscious; inappropriate response to environment [ex., vocalization, head pressing])	☐Drowsy/ Obtunded (↓ interaction with environment; slow response to verbal stimuli)	☐Stuporous (unresponsive unless aroused by noxious stimuli)	☐Coma (complete unresponsiveness to any stimuli)

- **Skin Elasticity**: ☐Normal skin turgor, ☐↓ Skin turgor, ☐Skin tent, ☐Gelatinous

- **Mucus Membranes**:
  - *CRT*:_____ [*RI*: 1–2; <1 = compensated shock, sepsis, heat stroke; <2 = acute decompensated shock; >2 = late decompensated shock, decreased cardiac output, hypothermia]
  - *Color*:_____ [*RI*: pink; red = compensated shock, sepsis, heat stroke; pale/white = anemia, shock; blue = cyanosis; yellow = hepatic disease, extravascular hemolysis; brown = met-Hb]
  - *Texture*:_____ [*RI*: moist = hydrated; tacky-to-dry = 5–12% dehydrated]

Physical Exam – Systems Checklist:

- **Head:** _____ ☐NAF
  - ○ Ears: ☐Ceruminous debris (mild / mod / sev) (AS / AD / AU), _____ ☐NAF
  - ○ Eyes: _____ ☐NAF
    - ▪ Retinal: _____ ☐NAF

→ Ⓛ	Ⓡ	Ⓛ	Ⓡ ←
☐ ⊙ Normal Direct	☐ ⊙ Normal Indirect	☐ ⊙ Normal Indirect	☐ ⊙ Normal Direct
☐ ⦿ Abnormal Direct	☐ ⦿ Abnormal Indirect	☐ ⦿ Abnormal Indirect	☐ ⦿ Abnormal Direct

  - ○ Nose: _____ ☐NAF
  - ○ Oral cavity: ☐Tarter/Gingivitis (mild / mod / sev), _____ ☐NAF
  - ○ Mandibular lnn.: ☐Enlarged Lt., ☐Enlarged Rt., _____ ☐NAF

- **Neck:** _____ ☐NAF
  - ○ Superficial cervical lnn.: ☐Enlarged Lt., ☐Enlarged Rt., _____ ☐NAF
  - ○ Thyroid: _____ ☐NAF

- **Thoracic limb:** _____ ☐NAF
  - ○ Foot pads: _____ ☐NAF
  - ○ Knuckling: _____ ☐NAF
  - ○ Axillary lnn. [normally absent]: _____ ☐NAF

- **Thorax:** _____ ☐NAF

- **Abdomen:** _____ ☐NAF
  - ○ Mammary chain: _____ ☐NAF
  - ○ Penis/ Testicles/ Vulva: _____ ☐NAF
  - ○ Superficial inguinal lnn. [normally absent]: _____ ☐NAF

- **Pelvic limb:** _____ ☐NAF
  - ○ Foot pads: _____ ☐NAF
  - ○ Knuckling: _____ ☐NAF
  - ○ Popliteal lnn.: ☐Enlarged Lt., ☐Enlarged Rt., _____ ☐NAF

- **Skin:** _____ ☐NAF
- **Tail:** _____ ☐NAF
- **Rectal☞⊙:** _____ ☐NAF

Problems List:

- **Problem #1**:

- **Problem #2**:

- **Problem #3**:

- **Problem #4**:

- **Problem #5**:

- **Problem #6**:

Diagnostic Plan	Treatment Plan

Case No._____

Patient	Age	Sex		Breed	Weight
		nM	sF		
	DOB:	iM	iF	Color:	kg

Owner	Primary Veterinarian	Admit Date/ Time
Name: Phone:	Name: Phone:	Date: Time: AM / PM

• **Presenting complaint**:_____
_____
_____
_____
_____
_____

• **Medical Hx**:_____
_____
_____
_____
_____

• **When/ where obtained**: Date:_____; ☐Breeder, ☐Shelter, Other:_____

Drug/ Supplement	Amount	Dose (mg/kg)	Route	Frequency	Date Started

• **Vaccine status – Dog**: ☐Rab ☐Parv ☐Dist ☐Aden; ☐Para ☐Lep ☐Bord ☐Influ ☐Lyme
• **Vaccine status – Cat**: ☐Rab ☐Herp ☐Cali ☐Pan ☐FeLV [kittens]; ☐FIV ☐Chlam ☐Bord
• **Heartworm / Flea & Tick / Intestinal Parasites**:
   ◦ *Last Heartworm Test*: Date:_____, ☐IDK; Test Results: ☐Pos, ☐Neg, ☐IDK
   ◦ *Monthly heartworm preventative*: ☐no ☐yes, Product:_____
   ◦ *Monthly flea & tick preventative*: ☐no ☐yes, Product:_____
   ◦ *Monthly dewormer*: ☐no ☐yes, Product:_____
• **Surgical Hx**: ☐Spay/Neuter; Date:_____; Other:_____
• **Environment**: ☐Indoor, ☐Outdoor, Time spent outdoors/ Other:_____
• **Housemates**: Dogs:_____ Cats:_____ Other:_____
• **Diet**: ☐Wet, ☐Dry; Brand/ Amt.:_____

Appetite	☐Normal, ☐↑, ☐↓
Weight	☐Normal, ☐↑, ☐↓; Past Wt.:_____ kg; Date:_____; Δ:_____
Thirst	☐Normal, ☐↑, ☐↓
Urination	☐Normal, ☐↑, ☐↓, ☐Blood, ☐Strain
Defecation	☐Normal, ☐↑, ☐↓, ☐Blood, ☐Strain, ☐Diarrhea, ☐Mucus
Discharge	☐No, ☐Yes; Onset/ Describe:
Cough/ Sneeze	☐No, ☐Yes; Onset/ Describe:
Vomit	☐No, ☐Yes; Onset/ Describe:
Respiration	☐Normal, ☐↑ Rate, ☐↑ Effort
Energy level	☐Normal, ☐Lethargic, ☐Exercise intolerance

• **Travel Hx**: ☐None, Other:_____
• **Exposure to**: ☐Standing water, ☐Wildlife, ☐Board/daycare, ☐Dog park, ☐Groomer, ☐Pet store
• **Adverse reactions to food/ meds**: ☐None, Other:_____
• **Can give oral meds**: ☐no ☐yes; Helpful Tricks:_____

Physical Exam – General:

- **Body Weight:**_____kg   **Body Condition Score:**___/9

- **Temperature:**_____°F [*Dog-RI*: 100.9–102.4; *Cat-RI*: 98.1–102.1]

- **Heart:**
  - *Rate:*_____beats/min [Dog-RI: 60–180; Cat-RI: 140–240 (in hospital)]
  - *Rhythm:* ☐Regular, ☐Irregular
  - *Sounds:* ☐None, ☐Split sound[S1 or S2], ☐Gallop[S3 or S4], ☐Murmur, ☐Muffled
    - *Grade:* ☐1–2[soft, only at PMI],   ☐3–4[moderate, mild radiate],   ☐5–6[loud, strong radiate, thrill]
    - *Timing:* ☐Systolic, ☐Diastolic, ☐Continuous
    - *PMI:*

	PMI	Over	Anatomic Boundaries
☐	Lt. apex	Mitral valve	5th to 6th ICS at level of CCJ
☐	Lt. base	Ao + Pul outflow	2nd to 4th ICS above the CCJ
☐	Rt. midheart	Tricuspid valve	3rd to 5th ICS near the CCJ
☐	Rt. sternal border	Right ventricle	5th to 7th ICS immediately dorsal to the sternum
☐	Sternal (cat)	Sternum	In cats, determination of PMI offers very little clinical significance.

  - *Vertebral Heart Size:* Dog = 8.7–10.7; Cat = 6.9–8.1 (from cranial edge of T4)
  - *Innocent Murmur:* Grade 1-2, systolic, left base location, disappear by ~4 months of age, absent clinical signs

- **Pulses:**
  - *Pulse rate:*_____pulses/min
  - *Character:*   ☐Sync, ☐Async;   ☐Normokinetic, ☐Hyper-, ☐Hypo-, ☐Variable

- **Lungs:**
  - *Respiratory rate:*_____breaths/min [*RI*: 16–30]
  - *Depth/Effort:* ☐Norm, ☐Pant, ☐Deep, ☐Shallow, ☐↑ Insp. effort, ☐↑ Exp. effort
  - *Sounds/Localization:*
    - ☐Norm BV, ☐Quiet BV, ☐Loud BV, ☐Crack, ☐Wheez, ☐Frict, ☐Muffled
    - ☐All lung fields, ☐Rt cran, ☐Rt mid, ☐Rt caud, ☐Lt cran, ☐Lt mid, ☐Lt caud
  - *Tracheal Auscultation/ Palpation:* ☐Normal, Other:_____

- **Pain Score:**_____ / 5   Localization:_____

- **Mentation:** ☐BAR   ☐Confused/   ☐Drowsy/   ☐Stuporous   ☐Coma
  ☐QAR   Disoriented   Obtunded   (unresponsive unless   (complete
  ☐Dull   (conscious; inappropriate   (↓ interaction with   aroused by noxious   unresponsiveness
  (conscious; responds   response to environment   environment; slow   stimuli)   to any stimuli)
  to sensory stimuli)   [ex., vocalization, head   response to verbal
  pressing])   stimuli)

- **Skin Elasticity:** ☐Normal skin turgor, ☐↓ Skin turgor, ☐Skin tent, ☐Gelatinous

- **Mucus Membranes:**
  - *CRT:*_____ [*RI*: 1–2; <1 = compensated shock, sepsis, heat stroke; <2 = acute decompensated shock; >2 = late decompensated shock, decreased cardiac output, hypothermia]
  - *Color:*_____ [*RI*: pink; red = compensated shock, sepsis, heat stroke; pale/white = anemia, shock; blue = cyanosis; yellow = hepatic disease, extravascular hemolysis; brown = met-Hb]
  - *Texture:*_____ [*RI*: moist = hydrated; tacky-to-dry = 5–12% dehydrated]

Physical Exam – Systems Checklist:

- Head:_____ ☐NAF
  - Ears: ☐Ceruminous debris (mild / mod / sev) (AS / AD / AU), _____ ☐NAF
  - Eyes:_____ ☐NAF
    - Retinal:_____ ☐NAF

→ Ⓛ		Ⓡ		Ⓛ		Ⓡ ←	
☐ ⊙ Normal Direct	☐ ⊙ Normal Indirect	☐ ⊙ Normal Indirect	☐ ⊙ Normal Direct
☐ ⊙ Abnormal Direct	☐ ⊙ Abnormal Indirect	☐ ⊙ Abnormal Indirect	☐ ⊙ Abnormal Direct

  - Nose:_____ ☐NAF
  - Oral cavity: ☐Tarter/Gingivitis (mild / mod / sev), _____ ☐NAF
  - Mandibular lnn.: ☐Enlarged Lt., ☐Enlarged Rt., _____ ☐NAF

- Neck:_____ ☐NAF
  - Superficial cervical lnn.: ☐Enlarged Lt., ☐Enlarged Rt., _____ ☐NAF
  - Thyroid:_____ ☐NAF

- Thoracic limb:_____ ☐NAF
  - Foot pads:_____ ☐NAF
  - Knuckling:_____ ☐NAF
  - Axillary lnn. [normally absent]:_____ ☐NAF

- Thorax:_____ ☐NAF

- Abdomen:_____ ☐NAF
  - Mammary chain:_____ ☐NAF
  - Penis/ Testicles/ Vulva:_____ ☐NAF
  - Superficial inguinal lnn. [normally absent]:_____ ☐NAF

- Pelvic limb:_____ ☐NAF
  - Foot pads:_____ ☐NAF
  - Knuckling:_____ ☐NAF
  - Popliteal lnn.: ☐Enlarged Lt., ☐Enlarged Rt., _____ ☐NAF

- Skin:_____ ☐NAF
- Tail:_____ ☐NAF
- Rectal☞⊙:_____ ☐NAF

Problems List:

• **Problem #1**:

• **Problem #2**:

• **Problem #3**:

• **Problem #4**:

• **Problem #5**:

• **Problem #6**:

Diagnostic Plan	Treatment Plan

Case No._____

Patient	Age	Sex		Breed	Weight
		nM	sF		
	DOB:	iM	iF	Color:	kg

Owner	Primary Veterinarian	Admit Date/ Time
Name: Phone:	Name: Phone:	Date: Time:　　　AM / PM

• **Presenting complaint**:_____
_____
_____
_____
_____
_____

• **Medical Hx**:_____
_____
_____
_____
_____

• **When/ where obtained**: Date:_____; □Breeder, □Shelter, Other:_____

Drug/ Supplement	Amount	Dose (mg/kg)	Route	Frequency	Date Started

• **Vaccine status – Dog**: □Rab □Parv □Dist □Aden; □Para □Lep □Bord □Influ □Lyme
• **Vaccine status – Cat**: □Rab □Herp □Cali □Pan □FeLV [kittens]; □FIV □Chlam □Bord
• **Heartworm / Flea & Tick / Intestinal Parasites**:
  ◦ *Last Heartworm Test*: Date:_____, □IDK; Test Results: □Pos, □Neg, □IDK
  ◦ *Monthly heartworm preventative*: □no □yes, Product:_____
  ◦ *Monthly flea & tick preventative*: □no □yes, Product:_____
  ◦ *Monthly dewormer*:　　　　　□no □yes, Product:_____
• **Surgical Hx**: □Spay/Neuter; Date:_____; Other:_____
• **Environment**: □Indoor, □Outdoor, Time spent outdoors/ Other:_____
• **Housemates**: Dogs:_____ Cats:_____ Other:_____
• **Diet**: □Wet, □Dry; Brand/ Amt.:_____

Appetite	□Normal, □↑, □↓
Weight	□Normal, □↑, □↓; Past Wt.:_____ kg; Date:_____; Δ:_____
Thirst	□Normal, □↑, □↓
Urination	□Normal, □↑, □↓, □Blood, □Strain
Defecation	□Normal, □↑, □↓, □Blood, □Strain, □Diarrhea, □Mucus
Discharge	□No, □Yes; Onset/ Describe:
Cough/ Sneeze	□No, □Yes; Onset/ Describe:
Vomit	□No, □Yes; Onset/ Describe:
Respiration	□Normal, □↑ Rate, □↑ Effort
Energy level	□Normal, □Lethargic, □Exercise intolerance

• **Travel Hx**: □None, Other:_____
• **Exposure to**: □Standing water, □Wildlife, □Board/daycare, □Dog park, □Groomer, □Pet store
• **Adverse reactions to food/ meds**: □None, Other:_____
• **Can give oral meds**: □no □yes; Helpful Tricks:_____

Physical Exam – General:

- **Body Weight:**_____kg   **Body Condition Score:**___/9

- **Temperature:**_____°F [*Dog-RI*: 100.9–102.4; *Cat-RI*: 98.1–102.1]

- **Heart**:
  - *Rate*:_____beats/min [Dog-RI: 60–180; Cat-RI: 140–240 (in hospital)]
  - *Rhythm*: □Regular, □Irregular
  - *Sounds*: □None, □Split sound[S1 or S2], □Gallop[S3 or S4], □Murmur, □Muffled
    - *Grade*: □1–2[soft, only at PMI], □3–4[moderate, mild radiate], □5–6[loud, strong radiate, thrill]
    - *Timing*: □Systolic, □Diastolic, □Continuous
    - *PMI*:

	PMI	Over	Anatomic Boundaries
□	Lt. apex	Mitral valve	5th to 6th ICS at level of CCJ
□	Lt. base	Ao + Pul outflow	2nd to 4th ICS above the CCJ
□	Rt. midheart	Tricuspid valve	3rd to 5th ICS near the CCJ
□	Rt. sternal border	Right ventricle	5th to 7th ICS immediately dorsal to the sternum
□	Sternal (cat)	Sternum	In cats, determination of PMI offers very little clinical significance.

  - • *Vertebral Heart Size*: Dog = 8.7–10.7; Cat = 6.9–8.1 (from cranial edge of T4)
  - • *Innocent Murmur*: Grade 1-2, systolic, left base location, disappear by ~4 months of age, absent clinical signs

- **Pulses**:
  - *Pulse rate*:_____pulses/min
  - *Character*: □Sync, □Async; □Normokinetic, □Hyper-, □Hypo-, □Variable

- **Lungs**:
  - *Respiratory rate*:_____breaths/min [*RI*: 16–30]
  - *Depth/Effort*: □Norm, □Pant, □Deep, □Shallow, □↑ Insp. effort, □↑ Exp. effort
  - *Sounds/Localization*:
    - □Norm BV, □Quiet BV, □Loud BV, □Crack, □Wheez, □Frict, □Muffled
    - □All lung fields, □Rt cran, □Rt mid, □Rt caud, □Lt cran, □Lt mid, □Lt caud
  - *Tracheal Auscultation/ Palpation*: □Normal, Other:_____

- **Pain Score:**_____ / 5   Localization:_____

- **Mentation**: □BAR   □Confused/   □Drowsy/   □Stuporous   □Coma
                  □QAR   Disoriented   Obtunded   (unresponsive unless   (complete
                  □Dull   (conscious; inappropriate   (↓ interaction with   aroused by noxious   unresponsiveness
                  (conscious; responds   response to environment   environment; slow   stimuli)   to any stimuli)
                  to sensory stimuli)   [ex., vocalization, head   response to verbal
                                    pressing])   stimuli)

- **Skin Elasticity**: □Normal skin turgor, □↓ Skin turgor, □Skin tent, □Gelatinous

- **Mucus Membranes**:
  - *CRT*:_____ [*RI*: 1–2; <1 = compensated shock, sepsis, heat stroke; <2 = acute decompensated shock; >2 = late decompensated shock, decreased cardiac output, hypothermia]
  - *Color*:_____ [*RI*: pink; red = compensated shock, sepsis, heat stroke; pale/white = anemia, shock; blue = cyanosis; yellow = hepatic disease, extravascular hemolysis; brown = met-Hb]
  - *Texture*:_____ [*RI*: moist = hydrated; tacky-to-dry = 5–12% dehydrated]

Physical Exam – Systems Checklist:

- Head:_____ ☐NAF
  - ○ Ears: ☐Ceruminous debris (mild / mod / sev) (AS / AD / AU),_____ ☐NAF
  - ○ Eyes:_____ ☐NAF
    - ▪ Retinal:_____ ☐NAF

→ ⓛ		ⓡ		ⓛ		ⓡ ←	
☐ ⊙ Normal Direct	☐ ⊙ Normal Indirect	☐ ⊙ Normal Indirect	☐ ⊙ Normal Direct
☐ ⊙ Abnormal Direct	☐ ⊙ Abnormal Indirect	☐ ⊙ Abnormal Indirect	☐ ⊙ Abnormal Direct

  - ○ Nose:_____ ☐NAF
  - ○ Oral cavity: ☐Tarter/Gingivitis (mild / mod / sev),_____ ☐NAF
  - ○ Mandibular lnn.: ☐Enlarged Lt., ☐Enlarged Rt.,_____ ☐NAF

- Neck:_____ ☐NAF
  - ○ Superficial cervical lnn.: ☐Enlarged Lt., ☐Enlarged Rt.,_____ ☐NAF
  - ○ Thyroid:_____ ☐NAF

- Thoracic limb:_____ ☐NAF
  - ○ Foot pads:_____ ☐NAF
  - ○ Knuckling:_____ ☐NAF
  - ○ Axillary lnn. [normally absent]:_____ ☐NAF

- Thorax:_____ ☐NAF

- Abdomen:_____ ☐NAF
  - ○ Mammary chain:_____ ☐NAF
  - ○ Penis/ Testicles/ Vulva:_____ ☐NAF
  - ○ Superficial inguinal lnn. [normally absent]:_____ ☐NAF

- Pelvic limb:_____ ☐NAF
  - ○ Foot pads:_____ ☐NAF
  - ○ Knuckling:_____ ☐NAF
  - ○ Popliteal lnn.: ☐Enlarged Lt., ☐Enlarged Rt.,_____ ☐NAF

- Skin:_____ ☐NAF
- Tail:_____ ☐NAF
- Rectal☞⊙:_____ ☐NAF

Problems List:

- **Problem #1**:

- **Problem #2**:

- **Problem #3**:

- **Problem #4**:

- **Problem #5**:

- **Problem #6**:

Diagnostic Plan	Treatment Plan

Case No._____

Patient	Age	Sex		Breed	Weight
		nM	sF		
	DOB:	iM	iF	Color:	kg

Owner	Primary Veterinarian	Admit Date/ Time
Name: Phone:	Name: Phone:	Date: Time: AM / PM

• **Presenting complaint**:_____
_____
_____
_____
_____
_____

• **Medical Hx**:_____
_____
_____
_____
_____

• **When/ where obtained**: Date:_____; ☐Breeder, ☐Shelter, Other:_____

Drug/ Supplement	Amount	Dose (mg/kg)	Route	Frequency	Date Started

• **Vaccine status – Dog**: ☐Rab ☐Parv ☐Dist ☐Aden; ☐Para ☐Lep ☐Bord ☐Influ ☐Lyme
• **Vaccine status – Cat**: ☐Rab ☐Herp ☐Cali ☐Pan ☐FeLV [kittens]; ☐FIV ☐Chlam ☐Bord
• **Heartworm / Flea & Tick / Intestinal Parasites**:
  ◦ *Last Heartworm Test*: Date:_____, ☐IDK; Test Results: ☐Pos, ☐Neg, ☐IDK
  ◦ *Monthly heartworm preventative*: ☐no ☐yes, Product:_____
  ◦ *Monthly flea & tick preventative*: ☐no ☐yes, Product:_____
  ◦ *Monthly dewormer*:   ☐no ☐yes, Product:_____
• **Surgical Hx**: ☐Spay/Neuter; Date:_____; Other:_____
• **Environment**: ☐Indoor, ☐Outdoor, Time spent outdoors/ Other:_____
• **Housemates**: Dogs:_____ Cats:_____ Other:_____
• **Diet**: ☐Wet, ☐Dry; Brand/ Amt.:_____

Appetite	☐Normal, ☐↑, ☐↓
Weight	☐Normal, ☐↑, ☐↓; Past Wt.:_____ kg; Date:_____; Δ:_____
Thirst	☐Normal, ☐↑, ☐↓
Urination	☐Normal, ☐↑, ☐↓, ☐Blood, ☐Strain
Defecation	☐Normal, ☐↑, ☐↓, ☐Blood, ☐Strain, ☐Diarrhea, ☐Mucus
Discharge	☐No, ☐Yes; Onset/ Describe:
Cough/ Sneeze	☐No, ☐Yes; Onset/ Describe:
Vomit	☐No, ☐Yes; Onset/ Describe:
Respiration	☐Normal, ☐↑ Rate, ☐↑ Effort
Energy level	☐Normal, ☐Lethargic, ☐Exercise intolerance

• **Travel Hx**: ☐None, Other:_____
• **Exposure to**: ☐Standing water, ☐Wildlife, ☐Board/daycare, ☐Dog park, ☐Groomer, ☐Pet store
• **Adverse reactions to food/ meds**: ☐None, Other:_____
• **Can give oral meds**: ☐no ☐yes; Helpful Tricks:_____

Physical Exam – General:

- **Body Weight**:_____kg   **Body Condition Score**:___/9

- **Temperature**:_____°F [*Dog-RI*: 100.9–102.4; *Cat-RI*: 98.1–102.1]

- **Heart**:
  - *Rate*:_____beats/min [Dog-RI: 60–180; Cat-RI: 140–240 (in hospital)]
  - *Rhythm*: ☐Regular, ☐Irregular
  - *Sounds*: ☐None, ☐Split sound[S1 or S2], ☐Gallop[S3 or S4], ☐Murmur, ☐Muffled
    - *Grade*: ☐1–2[soft, only at PMI],   ☐3–4[moderate, mild radiate],   ☐5–6[loud, strong radiate, thrill]
    - *Timing*: ☐Systolic, ☐Diastolic, ☐Continuous
    - *PMI*:

	PMI	Over	Anatomic Boundaries
☐	Lt. apex	Mitral valve	5th to 6th ICS at level of CCJ
☐	Lt. base	Ao + Pul outflow	2nd to 4th ICS above the CCJ
☐	Rt. midheart	Tricuspid valve	3rd to 5th ICS near the CCJ
☐	Rt. sternal border	Right ventricle	5th to 7th ICS immediately dorsal to the sternum
☐	Sternal (cat)	Sternum	In cats, determination of PMI offers very little clinical significance.

  - • *Vertebral Heart Size*: Dog = 8.7–10.7; Cat = 6.9–8.1 (from cranial edge of T4)
  - • *Innocent Murmur*: Grade 1-2, systolic, left base location, disappear by ~4 months of age, absent clinical signs

- **Pulses**:
  - *Pulse rate*:_____pulses/min
  - *Character*:   ☐Sync, ☐Async;   ☐Normokinetic, ☐Hyper-, ☐Hypo-, ☐Variable

- **Lungs**:
  - *Respiratory rate*:_____breaths/min [*RI*: 16–30]
  - *Depth/Effort*: ☐Norm, ☐Pant, ☐Deep, ☐Shallow, ☐↑ Insp. effort, ☐↑ Exp. effort
  - *Sounds/Localization*:
    - ☐Norm BV, ☐Quiet BV, ☐Loud BV, ☐Crack, ☐Wheez, ☐Frict, ☐Muffled
    - ☐All lung fields, ☐Rt cran, ☐Rt mid, ☐Rt caud, ☐Lt cran, ☐Lt mid, ☐Lt caud
  - *Tracheal Auscultation/ Palpation*: ☐Normal, Other:_____

- **Pain Score**:_____ / 5   Localization:_____

- **Mentation**:

☐BAR ☐QAR ☐Dull (conscious; responds to sensory stimuli)	☐Confused/ Disoriented (conscious; inappropriate response to environment [ex., vocalization, head pressing])	☐Drowsy/ Obtunded (↓ interaction with environment; slow response to verbal stimuli)	☐Stuporous (unresponsive unless aroused by noxious stimuli)	☐Coma (complete unresponsiveness to any stimuli)

- **Skin Elasticity**: ☐Normal skin turgor, ☐↓ Skin turgor, ☐Skin tent, ☐Gelatinous

- **Mucus Membranes**:
  - *CRT*:_____ [*RI*: 1–2; <1 = compensated shock, sepsis, heat stroke; <2 = acute decompensated shock; >2 = late decompensated shock, decreased cardiac output, hypothermia]
  - *Color*:_____ [*RI*: pink; red = compensated shock, sepsis, heat stroke; pale/white = anemia, shock; blue = cyanosis; yellow = hepatic disease, extravascular hemolysis; brown = met-Hb]
  - *Texture*:_____ [*RI*: moist = hydrated; tacky-to-dry = 5–12% dehydrated]

Physical Exam – Systems Checklist:

- Head: _____ ☐NAF
  - ◦ Ears: ☐Ceruminous debris (mild / mod / sev) (AS / AD / AU), _____ ☐NAF
  - ◦ Eyes: _____ ☐NAF
    - ▪ Retinal: _____ ☐NAF

→ Ⓛ		Ⓡ		Ⓛ		Ⓡ ←	
☐ ⊙ Normal Direct		☐ ⊙ Normal Indirect		☐ ⊙ Normal Indirect		☐ ⊙ Normal Direct	
☐ ● Abnormal Direct		☐ ● Abnormal Indirect		☐ ● Abnormal Indirect		☐ ● Abnormal Direct	

  - ◦ Nose: _____ ☐NAF
  - ◦ Oral cavity: ☐Tarter/Gingivitis (mild / mod / sev), _____ ☐NAF
  - ◦ Mandibular lnn.: ☐Enlarged Lt., ☐Enlarged Rt., _____ ☐NAF

- Neck: _____ ☐NAF
  - ◦ Superficial cervical lnn.: ☐Enlarged Lt., ☐Enlarged Rt., _____ ☐NAF
  - ◦ Thyroid: _____ ☐NAF

- Thoracic limb: _____ ☐NAF
  - ◦ Foot pads: _____ ☐NAF
  - ◦ Knuckling: _____ ☐NAF
  - ◦ Axillary lnn. [normally absent]: _____ ☐NAF

- Thorax: _____ ☐NAF

- Abdomen: _____ ☐NAF
  - ◦ Mammary chain: _____ ☐NAF
  - ◦ Penis/ Testicles/ Vulva: _____ ☐NAF
  - ◦ Superficial inguinal lnn. [normally absent]: _____ ☐NAF

- Pelvic limb: _____ ☐NAF
  - ◦ Foot pads: _____ ☐NAF
  - ◦ Knuckling: _____ ☐NAF
  - ◦ Popliteal lnn.: ☐Enlarged Lt., ☐Enlarged Rt., _____ ☐NAF

- Skin: _____ ☐NAF
- Tail: _____ ☐NAF
- Rectal☞⊙: _____ ☐NAF

Problems List:

- **Problem #1**:

- **Problem #2**:

- **Problem #3**:

- **Problem #4**:

- **Problem #5**:

- **Problem #6**:

Diagnostic Plan	Treatment Plan

Case No._____

Patient	Age	Sex		Breed		Weight
		nM	sF			
	DOB:	iM	iF	Color:		kg

Owner	Primary Veterinarian	Admit Date/ Time
Name: Phone:	Name: Phone:	Date: Time: AM / PM

• Presenting complaint:_____
_____
_____
_____
_____
_____
_____

• Medical Hx:_____
_____
_____
_____
_____

• When/ where obtained: Date:_____; □Breeder, □Shelter, Other:_____

Drug/ Supplement	Amount	Dose (mg/kg)	Route	Frequency	Date Started

• Vaccine status – Dog: □Rab □Parv □Dist □Aden; □Para □Lep □Bord □Influ □Lyme
• Vaccine status – Cat: □Rab □Herp □Cali □Pan □FeLV [kittens]; □FIV □Chlam □Bord
• Heartworm / Flea & Tick / Intestinal Parasites:
   ◦ *Last Heartworm Test*: Date:_____, □IDK; Test Results: □Pos, □Neg, □IDK
   ◦ *Monthly heartworm preventative*: □no □yes, Product:_____
   ◦ *Monthly flea & tick preventative*: □no □yes, Product:_____
   ◦ *Monthly dewormer*:   □no □yes, Product:_____
• Surgical Hx: □Spay/Neuter; Date:_____; Other:_____
• Environment: □Indoor, □Outdoor, Time spent outdoors/ Other:_____
• Housemates: Dogs:_____ Cats:_____ Other:_____
• Diet: □Wet, □Dry; Brand/ Amt.:_____

Appetite	□Normal, □↑, □↓
Weight	□Normal, □↑, □↓; Past Wt.:_____ kg; Date:_____; Δ:_____
Thirst	□Normal, □↑, □↓
Urination	□Normal, □↑, □↓, □Blood, □Strain
Defecation	□Normal, □↑, □↓, □Blood, □Strain, □Diarrhea, □Mucus
Discharge	□No, □Yes; Onset/ Describe:
Cough/ Sneeze	□No, □Yes; Onset/ Describe:
Vomit	□No, □Yes; Onset/ Describe:
Respiration	□Normal, □↑ Rate, □↑ Effort
Energy level	□Normal, □Lethargic, □Exercise intolerance

• Travel Hx: □None, Other:_____
• Exposure to: □Standing water, □Wildlife, □Board/daycare, □Dog park, □Groomer, □Pet store
• Adverse reactions to food/ meds: □None, Other:_____
• Can give oral meds: □no □yes; Helpful Tricks:_____

<u>Physical Exam – General</u>:

- **Body Weight**:_____kg   **Body Condition Score**:___/9

- **Temperature**:_____°F [*Dog-RI*: 100.9–102.4;   *Cat-RI*: 98.1–102.1]

- **Heart**:
  - *Rate*:_____beats/min [Dog-RI: 60–180;   Cat-RI: 140–240 (in hospital)]
  - *Rhythm*: ☐Regular, ☐Irregular
  - *Sounds*: ☐None, ☐Split sound[S1 or S2], ☐Gallop[S3 or S4], ☐Murmur, ☐Muffled
    - *Grade*: ☐1–2[soft, only at PMI],   ☐3–4[moderate, mild radiate],   ☐5–6[loud, strong radiate, thrill]
    - *Timing*: ☐Systolic, ☐Diastolic, ☐Continuous
    - *PMI*:

	PMI	Over	Anatomic Boundaries
☐	Lt. apex	Mitral valve	5th to 6th ICS at level of CCJ
☐	Lt. base	Ao + Pul outflow	2nd to 4th ICS above the CCJ
☐	Rt. midheart	Tricuspid valve	3rd to 5th ICS near the CCJ
☐	Rt. sternal border	Right ventricle	5th to 7th ICS immediately dorsal to the sternum
☐	Sternal (cat)	Sternum	In cats, determination of PMI offers very little clinical significance.

  - •   *Vertebral Heart Size*: Dog = 8.7–10.7; Cat = 6.9–8.1 (from cranial edge of T4)
  - •   *Innocent Murmur*: Grade 1-2, systolic, left base location, disappear by ~4 months of age, absent clinical signs

- **Pulses**:
  - *Pulse rate*:_____pulses/min
  - *Character*:   ☐Sync, ☐Async;   ☐Normokinetic, ☐Hyper-, ☐Hypo-, ☐Variable

- **Lungs**:
  - *Respiratory rate*:_____breaths/min [*RI*: 16–30]
  - *Depth/Effort*: ☐Norm, ☐Pant, ☐Deep, ☐Shallow, ☐↑ Insp. effort, ☐↑ Exp. effort
  - *Sounds/Localization*:
    - ☐Norm BV, ☐Quiet BV, ☐Loud BV, ☐Crack, ☐Wheez, ☐Frict, ☐Muffled
    - ☐All lung fields, ☐Rt cran, ☐Rt mid, ☐Rt caud, ☐Lt cran, ☐Lt mid, ☐Lt caud
  - *Tracheal Auscultation/ Palpation*: ☐Normal, Other:_____

- **Pain Score**:_____ / 5   Localization:_____

- **Mentation**: ☐BAR   ☐Confused/   ☐Drowsy/   ☐Stuporous   ☐Coma
  - ☐QAR   Disoriented   Obtunded   (unresponsive unless   (complete
  - ☐Dull   (conscious; inappropriate   (↓ interaction with   aroused by noxious   unresponsiveness
  - (conscious; responds   response to environment   environment; slow   stimuli)   to any stimuli)
  - to sensory stimuli)   [ex., vocalization, head   response to verbal
  - pressing])   stimuli)

- **Skin Elasticity**: ☐Normal skin turgor,   ☐↓ Skin turgor, ☐Skin tent, ☐Gelatinous

- **Mucus Membranes**:
  - *CRT*:_____ [*RI*: 1–2; <1 = compensated shock, sepsis, heat stroke; <2 = acute decompensated shock; >2 = late decompensated shock, decreased cardiac output, hypothermia]
  - *Color*:_____ [*RI*: pink; red = compensated shock, sepsis, heat stroke; pale/white = anemia, shock; blue = cyanosis; yellow = hepatic disease, extravascular hemolysis; brown = met-Hb]
  - *Texture*:_____ [*RI*: moist = hydrated; tacky-to-dry = 5–12% dehydrated]

Physical Exam – Systems Checklist:

- Head:_____ ☐NAF
  - ○ Ears: ☐Ceruminous debris (mild / mod / sev) (AS / AD / AU), _____ ☐NAF
  - ○ Eyes:_____ ☐NAF
    - ▪ Retinal:_____ ☐NAF

→ Ⓛ		Ⓡ		Ⓛ		Ⓡ ←	
☐	⊙ Normal Direct	☐	⊙ Normal Indirect	☐	⊙ Normal Indirect	☐	⊙ Normal Direct
☐	⊙ Abnormal Direct	☐	⊙ Abnormal Indirect	☐	⊙ Abnormal Indirect	☐	⊙ Abnormal Direct

  - ○ Nose:_____ ☐NAF
  - ○ Oral cavity: ☐Tarter/Gingivitis (mild / mod / sev), _____ ☐NAF
  - ○ Mandibular lnn.: ☐Enlarged Lt., ☐Enlarged Rt., _____ ☐NAF

- Neck:_____ ☐NAF
  - ○ Superficial cervical lnn.: ☐Enlarged Lt., ☐Enlarged Rt., _____ ☐NAF
  - ○ Thyroid:_____ ☐NAF

- Thoracic limb:_____ ☐NAF
  - ○ Foot pads:_____ ☐NAF
  - ○ Knuckling:_____ ☐NAF
  - ○ Axillary lnn. [normally absent]:_____ ☐NAF

- Thorax:_____ ☐NAF

- Abdomen:_____ ☐NAF
  - ○ Mammary chain:_____ ☐NAF
  - ○ Penis/ Testicles/ Vulva:_____ ☐NAF
  - ○ Superficial inguinal lnn. [normally absent]:_____ ☐NAF

- Pelvic limb:_____ ☐NAF
  - ○ Foot pads:_____ ☐NAF
  - ○ Knuckling:_____ ☐NAF
  - ○ Popliteal lnn.: ☐Enlarged Lt., ☐Enlarged Rt., _____ ☐NAF

- Skin:_____ ☐NAF
- Tail:_____ ☐NAF
- Rectal☞☉:_____ ☐NAF

Problems List:

- **Problem #1**:

- **Problem #2**:

- **Problem #3**:

- **Problem #4**:

- **Problem #5**:

- **Problem #6**:

Diagnostic Plan	Treatment Plan

Case No._____

Patient	Age	Sex		Breed	Weight
		nM	sF		
	DOB:	iM	iF	Color:	kg

Owner		Primary Veterinarian	Admit Date/ Time
Name: Phone:		Name: Phone:	Date: Time: AM / PM

• **Presenting complaint**:_____
_____
_____
_____
_____
_____

• **Medical Hx**:_____
_____
_____
_____
_____

• **When/ where obtained**: Date:_____; ☐Breeder, ☐Shelter, Other:_____

Drug/ Supplement	Amount	Dose (mg/kg)	Route	Frequency	Date Started

• **Vaccine status – Dog**: ☐Rab ☐Parv ☐Dist ☐Aden; ☐Para ☐Lep ☐Bord ☐Influ ☐Lyme
• **Vaccine status – Cat**: ☐Rab ☐Herp ☐Cali ☐Pan ☐FeLV [kittens]; ☐FIV ☐Chlam ☐Bord
• **Heartworm / Flea & Tick / Intestinal Parasites**:
  ◦ *Last Heartworm Test*: Date:_____, ☐IDK; Test Results: ☐Pos, ☐Neg, ☐IDK
  ◦ *Monthly heartworm preventative*: ☐no ☐yes, Product:_____
  ◦ *Monthly flea & tick preventative*: ☐no ☐yes, Product:_____
  ◦ *Monthly dewormer*:   ☐no ☐yes, Product:_____
• **Surgical Hx**: ☐Spay/Neuter; Date:_____; Other:_____
• **Environment**: ☐Indoor, ☐Outdoor, Time spent outdoors/ Other:_____
• **Housemates**: Dogs:_____ Cats:_____ Other:_____
• **Diet**: ☐Wet, ☐Dry; Brand/ Amt.:_____

Appetite	☐Normal, ☐↑, ☐↓
Weight	☐Normal, ☐↑, ☐↓; Past Wt.:_____ kg; Date:_____; Δ:_____
Thirst	☐Normal, ☐↑, ☐↓
Urination	☐Normal, ☐↑, ☐↓, ☐Blood, ☐Strain
Defecation	☐Normal, ☐↑, ☐↓, ☐Blood, ☐Strain, ☐Diarrhea, ☐Mucus
Discharge	☐No, ☐Yes; Onset/ Describe:
Cough/ Sneeze	☐No, ☐Yes; Onset/ Describe:
Vomit	☐No, ☐Yes; Onset/ Describe:
Respiration	☐Normal, ☐↑ Rate, ☐↑ Effort
Energy level	☐Normal, ☐Lethargic, ☐Exercise intolerance

• **Travel Hx**: ☐None, Other:_____
• **Exposure to**: ☐Standing water, ☐Wildlife, ☐Board/daycare, ☐Dog park, ☐Groomer, ☐Pet store
• **Adverse reactions to food/ meds**: ☐None, Other:_____
• **Can give oral meds**: ☐no ☐yes; Helpful Tricks:_____

Physical Exam – General:

- **Body Weight**:_____kg   **Body Condition Score**:____/9

- **Temperature**:_____°F [*Dog-RI*: 100.9–102.4; *Cat-RI*: 98.1–102.1]

- **Heart**:
    - *Rate*:_____beats/min [Dog-RI: 60–180; Cat-RI: 140–240 (in hospital)]
    - *Rhythm*: ☐Regular, ☐Irregular
    - *Sounds*: ☐None, ☐Split sound[S1 or S2], ☐Gallop[S3 or S4], ☐Murmur, ☐Muffled
        - *Grade*: ☐1–2[soft, only at PMI], ☐3–4[moderate, mild radiate], ☐5–6[loud, strong radiate, thrill]
        - *Timing*: ☐Systolic, ☐Diastolic, ☐Continuous
        - *PMI*:

	PMI	Over	Anatomic Boundaries
☐	Lt. apex	Mitral valve	5th to 6th ICS at level of CCJ
☐	Lt. base	Ao + Pul outflow	2nd to 4th ICS above the CCJ
☐	Rt. midheart	Tricuspid valve	3rd to 5th ICS near the CCJ
☐	Rt. sternal border	Right ventricle	5th to 7th ICS immediately dorsal to the sternum
☐	Sternal (cat)	Sternum	In cats, determination of PMI offers very little clinical significance.

- *Vertebral Heart Size*: Dog = 8.7–10.7; Cat = 6.9–8.1 (from cranial edge of T4)
- *Innocent Murmur*: Grade 1-2, systolic, left base location, disappear by ~4 months of age, absent clinical signs

- **Pulses**:
    - *Pulse rate*:_____pulses/min
    - *Character*: ☐Sync, ☐Async; ☐Normokinetic, ☐Hyper-, ☐Hypo-, ☐Variable

- **Lungs**:
    - *Respiratory rate*:_____breaths/min [*RI*: 16–30]
    - *Depth/Effort*: ☐Norm, ☐Pant, ☐Deep, ☐Shallow, ☐↑ Insp. effort, ☐↑ Exp. effort
    - *Sounds/Localization*:
        - ☐Norm BV, ☐Quiet BV, ☐Loud BV, ☐Crack, ☐Wheez, ☐Frict, ☐Muffled
        - ☐All lung fields, ☐Rt cran, ☐Rt mid, ☐Rt caud, ☐Lt cran, ☐Lt mid, ☐Lt caud
    - *Tracheal Auscultation/ Palpation*: ☐Normal, Other:_____

- **Pain Score**:_____ / 5   Localization:_____

- **Mentation**: ☐BAR   ☐Confused/   ☐Drowsy/   ☐Stuporous   ☐Coma
  ☐QAR   Disoriented   Obtunded   (unresponsive unless   (complete
  ☐Dull   (conscious; inappropriate   (↓ interaction with   aroused by noxious   unresponsiveness
  (conscious; responds   response to environment   environment; slow   stimuli)   to any stimuli)
  to sensory stimuli)   [ex., vocalization, head   response to verbal
  pressing])   stimuli)

- **Skin Elasticity**: ☐Normal skin turgor, ☐↓ Skin turgor, ☐Skin tent, ☐Gelatinous

- **Mucus Membranes**:
    - *CRT*:_____ [*RI*: 1–2; <1 = compensated shock, sepsis, heat stroke; <2 = acute decompensated shock;
      >2 = late decompensated shock, decreased cardiac output, hypothermia]
    - *Color*:_____ [*RI*: pink; red = compensated shock, sepsis, heat stroke; pale/white = anemia, shock;
      blue = cyanosis; yellow = hepatic disease, extravascular hemolysis; brown = met-Hb]
    - *Texture*:_____ [*RI*: moist = hydrated; tacky-to-dry = 5–12% dehydrated]

Physical Exam – Systems Checklist:

- Head: _____ ☐NAF
  - Ears: ☐Ceruminous debris (mild / mod / sev) (AS / AD / AU), _____ ☐NAF
  - Eyes: _____ ☐NAF
    - Retinal: _____ ☐NAF

→ Ⓛ		Ⓡ		Ⓛ		Ⓡ ←	
☐	◉ Normal Direct	☐	◉ Normal Indirect	☐	◉ Normal Indirect	☐	◉ Normal Direct
☐	◉ Abnormal Direct	☐	◉ Abnormal Indirect	☐	◉ Abnormal Indirect	☐	◉ Abnormal Direct

  - Nose: _____ ☐NAF
  - Oral cavity: ☐Tarter/Gingivitis (mild / mod / sev), _____ ☐NAF
  - Mandibular lnn.: ☐Enlarged Lt., ☐Enlarged Rt., _____ ☐NAF

- Neck: _____ ☐NAF
  - Superficial cervical lnn.: ☐Enlarged Lt., ☐Enlarged Rt., _____ ☐NAF
  - Thyroid: _____ ☐NAF

- Thoracic limb: _____ ☐NAF
  - Foot pads: _____ ☐NAF
  - Knuckling: _____ ☐NAF
  - Axillary lnn. [normally absent]: _____ ☐NAF

- Thorax: _____ ☐NAF

- Abdomen: _____ ☐NAF
  - Mammary chain: _____ ☐NAF
  - Penis/ Testicles/ Vulva: _____ ☐NAF
  - Superficial inguinal lnn. [normally absent]: _____ ☐NAF

- Pelvic limb: _____ ☐NAF
  - Foot pads: _____ ☐NAF
  - Knuckling: _____ ☐NAF
  - Popliteal lnn.: ☐Enlarged Lt., ☐Enlarged Rt., _____ ☐NAF

- Skin: _____ ☐NAF
- Tail: _____ ☐NAF
- Rectal☞☉: _____ ☐NAF

Problems List:

- **Problem #1**:

- **Problem #2**:

- **Problem #3**:

- **Problem #4**:

- **Problem #5**:

- **Problem #6**:

Diagnostic Plan	Treatment Plan

Case No._____

Patient	Age	Sex		Breed		Weight
		nM	sF			
	DOB:	iM	iF	Color:		kg

Owner	Primary Veterinarian	Admit Date/ Time
Name: Phone:	Name: Phone:	Date: Time: AM / PM

• **Presenting complaint**:_____
_____
_____
_____
_____
_____

• **Medical Hx**:_____
_____
_____
_____
_____

• **When/ where obtained**: Date:_____; □Breeder, □Shelter, Other:_____

Drug/ Supplement	Amount	Dose (mg/kg)	Route	Frequency	Date Started

• **Vaccine status – Dog**: □Rab □Parv □Dist □Aden; □Para □Lep □Bord □Influ □Lyme
• **Vaccine status – Cat**: □Rab □Herp □Cali □Pan □FeLV [kittens]; □FIV □Chlam □Bord
• **Heartworm / Flea & Tick / Intestinal Parasites**:
  ◦ *Last Heartworm Test*: Date:_____, □IDK; Test Results: □Pos, □Neg, □IDK
  ◦ *Monthly heartworm preventative*: □no □yes, Product:_____
  ◦ *Monthly flea & tick preventative*: □no □yes, Product:_____
  ◦ *Monthly dewormer*: □no □yes, Product:_____
• **Surgical Hx**: □Spay/Neuter; Date:_____; Other:_____
• **Environment**: □Indoor, □Outdoor, Time spent outdoors/ Other:_____
• **Housemates**: Dogs:_____ Cats:_____ Other:_____
• **Diet**: □Wet, □Dry; Brand/ Amt.:_____

Appetite	□Normal, □↑, □↓
Weight	□Normal, □↑, □↓; Past Wt.:_____ kg; Date:_____; Δ:_____
Thirst	□Normal, □↑, □↓
Urination	□Normal, □↑, □↓, □Blood, □Strain
Defecation	□Normal, □↑, □↓, □Blood, □Strain, □Diarrhea, □Mucus
Discharge	□No, □Yes; Onset/ Describe:
Cough/ Sneeze	□No, □Yes; Onset/ Describe:
Vomit	□No, □Yes; Onset/ Describe:
Respiration	□Normal, □↑ Rate, □↑ Effort
Energy level	□Normal, □Lethargic, □Exercise intolerance

• **Travel Hx**: □None, Other:_____
• **Exposure to**: □Standing water, □Wildlife, □Board/daycare, □Dog park, □Groomer, □Pet store
• **Adverse reactions to food/ meds**: □None, Other:_____
• **Can give oral meds**: □no □yes; Helpful Tricks:_____

Physical Exam – General:

- **Body Weight:**_____kg **Body Condition Score:**___/9

- **Temperature:**_____°F [*Dog-RI*: 100.9–102.4; *Cat-RI*: 98.1–102.1]

- **Heart**:
  - *Rate*:_____beats/min [Dog-RI: 60–180; Cat-RI: 140–240 (in hospital)]
  - *Rhythm*: □Regular, □Irregular
  - *Sounds*: □None, □Split sound[S1 or S2], □Gallop[S3 or S4], □Murmur, □Muffled
    - *Grade*: □1–2[soft, only at PMI], □3–4[moderate, mild radiate], □5–6[loud, strong radiate, thrill]
    - *Timing*: □Systolic, □Diastolic, □Continuous
    - *PMI*:

	PMI	Over	Anatomic Boundaries
□	Lt. apex	Mitral valve	5th to 6th ICS at level of CCJ
□	Lt. base	Ao + Pul outflow	2nd to 4th ICS above the CCJ
□	Rt. midheart	Tricuspid valve	3rd to 5th ICS near the CCJ
□	Rt. sternal border	Right ventricle	5th to 7th ICS immediately dorsal to the sternum
□	Sternal (cat)	Sternum	In cats, determination of PMI offers very little clinical significance.

  - *Vertebral Heart Size*: Dog = 8.7–10.7; Cat = 6.9–8.1 (from cranial edge of T4)
  - *Innocent Murmur*: Grade 1-2, systolic, left base location, disappear by ~4 months of age, absent clinical signs

- **Pulses**:
  - *Pulse rate*:_____pulses/min
  - *Character*: □Sync, □Async; □Normokinetic, □Hyper-, □Hypo-, □Variable

- **Lungs**:
  - *Respiratory rate*:_____breaths/min [*RI*: 16–30]
  - *Depth/Effort*: □Norm, □Pant, □Deep, □Shallow, □↑ Insp. effort, □↑ Exp. effort
  - *Sounds/Localization*:
    - □Norm BV, □Quiet BV, □Loud BV, □Crack, □Wheez, □Frict, □Muffled
    - □All lung fields, □Rt cran, □Rt mid, □Rt caud, □Lt cran, □Lt mid, □Lt caud
  - *Tracheal Auscultation/ Palpation*: □Normal, Other:_____

- **Pain Score**:_____ / 5   Localization:_____

- **Mentation**:

□BAR	□Confused/	□Drowsy/	□Stuporous	□Coma
□QAR	Disoriented	Obtunded	(unresponsive unless aroused by noxious stimuli)	(complete unresponsiveness to any stimuli)
□Dull	(conscious; inappropriate response to environment [ex., vocalization, head pressing])	(↓ interaction with environment; slow response to verbal stimuli)		
(conscious; responds to sensory stimuli)				

- **Skin Elasticity**: □Normal skin turgor, □↓ Skin turgor, □Skin tent, □Gelatinous

- **Mucus Membranes**:
  - *CRT*:_____ [*RI*: 1–2; <1 = compensated shock, sepsis, heat stroke; <2 = acute decompensated shock; >2 = late decompensated shock, decreased cardiac output, hypothermia]
  - *Color*:_____ [*RI*: pink; red = compensated shock, sepsis, heat stroke; pale/white = anemia, shock; blue = cyanosis; yellow = hepatic disease, extravascular hemolysis; brown = met-Hb]
  - *Texture*:_____ [*RI*: moist = hydrated; tacky-to-dry = 5–12% dehydrated]

Physical Exam – Systems Checklist:

- Head:_____ ☐NAF
  - Ears: ☐Ceruminous debris (mild / mod / sev) (AS / AD / AU), _____ ☐NAF
  - Eyes:_____ ☐NAF
    - Retinal:_____ ☐NAF

→ Ⓛ		Ⓡ		Ⓛ		Ⓡ ←	
☐	◉ Normal Direct	☐	◉ Normal Indirect	☐	◉ Normal Indirect	☐	◉ Normal Direct
☐	◉ Abnormal Direct	☐	● Abnormal Indirect	☐	● Abnormal Indirect	☐	● Abnormal Direct

  - Nose:_____ ☐NAF
  - Oral cavity: ☐Tarter/Gingivitis (mild / mod / sev), _____ ☐NAF
  - Mandibular lnn.: ☐Enlarged Lt., ☐Enlarged Rt., _____ ☐NAF

- Neck:_____ ☐NAF
  - Superficial cervical lnn.: ☐Enlarged Lt., ☐Enlarged Rt., _____ ☐NAF
  - Thyroid:_____ ☐NAF

- Thoracic limb:_____ ☐NAF
  - Foot pads:_____ ☐NAF
  - Knuckling:_____ ☐NAF
  - Axillary lnn. [normally absent]:_____ ☐NAF

- Thorax:_____ ☐NAF

- Abdomen:_____ ☐NAF
  - Mammary chain:_____ ☐NAF
  - Penis/ Testicles/ Vulva:_____ ☐NAF
  - Superficial inguinal lnn. [normally absent]:_____ ☐NAF

- Pelvic limb:_____ ☐NAF
  - Foot pads:_____ ☐NAF
  - Knuckling:_____ ☐NAF
  - Popliteal lnn.: ☐Enlarged Lt., ☐Enlarged Rt., _____ ☐NAF

- Skin:_____ ☐NAF
- Tail:_____ ☐NAF
- Rectal☞⊙:_____ ☐NAF

Problems List:

- **Problem #1**:

- **Problem #2**:

- **Problem #3**:

- **Problem #4**:

- **Problem #5**:

- **Problem #6**:

Diagnostic Plan	Treatment Plan

Case No._____

Patient	Age	Sex		Breed	Weight
		nM	sF		
	DOB:	iM	iF	Color:	kg

Owner	Primary Veterinarian	Admit Date/ Time
Name: Phone:	Name: Phone:	Date: Time: AM / PM

• Presenting complaint:_____
_____
_____
_____
_____
_____

• Medical Hx:_____
_____
_____
_____
_____

• When/ where obtained: Date:_____; □Breeder, □Shelter, Other:_____

Drug/ Supplement	Amount	Dose (mg/kg)	Route	Frequency	Date Started

• Vaccine status – Dog: □Rab □Parv □Dist □Aden; □Para □Lep □Bord □Influ □Lyme
• Vaccine status – Cat: □Rab □Herp □Cali □Pan □FeLV [kittens]; □FIV □Chlam □Bord
• Heartworm / Flea & Tick / Intestinal Parasites:
   ○ *Last Heartworm Test*: Date:_____, □IDK; Test Results: □Pos, □Neg, □IDK
   ○ *Monthly heartworm preventative*: □no □yes, Product:_____
   ○ *Monthly flea & tick preventative*: □no □yes, Product:_____
   ○ *Monthly dewormer*: □no □yes, Product:_____
• Surgical Hx: □Spay/Neuter; Date:_____; Other:_____
• Environment: □Indoor, □Outdoor, Time spent outdoors/ Other:_____
• Housemates: Dogs:_____ Cats:_____ Other:_____
• Diet: □Wet, □Dry; Brand/ Amt.:_____

Appetite	□Normal, □↑, □↓
Weight	□Normal, □↑, □↓; Past Wt.:_____ kg; Date:_____; Δ:_____
Thirst	□Normal, □↑, □↓
Urination	□Normal, □↑, □↓, □Blood, □Strain
Defecation	□Normal, □↑, □↓, □Blood, □Strain, □Diarrhea, □Mucus
Discharge	□No, □Yes; Onset/ Describe:
Cough/ Sneeze	□No, □Yes; Onset/ Describe:
Vomit	□No, □Yes; Onset/ Describe:
Respiration	□Normal, □↑ Rate, □↑ Effort
Energy level	□Normal, □Lethargic, □Exercise intolerance

• Travel Hx: □None, Other:_____
• Exposure to: □Standing water, □Wildlife, □Board/daycare, □Dog park, □Groomer, □Pet store
• Adverse reactions to food/ meds: □None, Other:_____
• Can give oral meds: □no □yes; Helpful Tricks:_____

Physical Exam – General:

- **Body Weight**:_____kg   **Body Condition Score**:___/9

- **Temperature**:_____°F [*Dog-RI*: 100.9–102.4; *Cat-RI*: 98.1–102.1]

- **Heart**:
  - *Rate*:_____beats/min [Dog-RI: 60–180; Cat-RI: 140–240 (in hospital)]
  - *Rhythm*: □Regular, □Irregular
  - *Sounds*: □None, □Split sound[S1 or S2], □Gallop[S3 or S4], □Murmur, □Muffled
    - *Grade*: □1–2[soft, only at PMI],   □3–4[moderate, mild radiate],   □5–6[loud, strong radiate, thrill]
    - *Timing*: □Systolic, □Diastolic, □Continuous
    - *PMI*:

	PMI	Over	Anatomic Boundaries
□	Lt. apex	Mitral valve	5th to 6th ICS at level of CCJ
□	Lt. base	Ao + Pul outflow	2nd to 4th ICS above the CCJ
□	Rt. midheart	Tricuspid valve	3rd to 5th ICS near the CCJ
□	Rt. sternal border	Right ventricle	5th to 7th ICS immediately dorsal to the sternum
□	Sternal (cat)	Sternum	In cats, determination of PMI offers very little clinical significance.

  - • *Vertebral Heart Size*: Dog = 8.7–10.7; Cat = 6.9–8.1 (from cranial edge of T4)
  - • *Innocent Murmur*: Grade 1-2, systolic, left base location, disappear by ~4 months of age, absent clinical signs

- **Pulses**:
  - *Pulse rate*:_____pulses/min
  - *Character*:   □Sync, □Async;   □Normokinetic, □Hyper-, □Hypo-, □Variable

- **Lungs**:
  - *Respiratory rate*:_____breaths/min [*RI*: 16–30]
  - *Depth/Effort*: □Norm, □Pant, □Deep, □Shallow, □↑ Insp. effort, □↑ Exp. effort
  - *Sounds/Localization*:
    - □Norm BV, □Quiet BV, □Loud BV, □Crack, □Wheez, □Frict, □Muffled
    - □All lung fields, □Rt cran, □Rt mid, □Rt caud, □Lt cran, □Lt mid, □Lt caud
  - *Tracheal Auscultation/ Palpation*: □Normal, Other:_____

- **Pain Score**:_____ / 5   Localization:_____

- **Mentation**: □BAR   □Confused/   □Drowsy/   □Stuporous   □Coma
              □QAR   Disoriented   Obtunded   (unresponsive unless   (complete
              □Dull   (conscious; inappropriate   (↓ interaction with   aroused by noxious   unresponsiveness
              (conscious; responds   response to environment   environment; slow   stimuli)   to any stimuli)
              to sensory stimuli)   [ex., vocalization, head   response to verbal
                                pressing])   stimuli)

- **Skin Elasticity**: □Normal skin turgor, □↓ Skin turgor, □Skin tent, □Gelatinous

- **Mucus Membranes**:
  - *CRT*:_____ [*RI*: 1–2; <1 = compensated shock, sepsis, heat stroke; <2 = acute decompensated shock; >2 = late decompensated shock, decreased cardiac output, hypothermia]
  - *Color*:_____ [*RI*: pink; red = compensated shock, sepsis, heat stroke; pale/white = anemia, shock; blue = cyanosis; yellow = hepatic disease, extravascular hemolysis; brown = met-Hb]
  - *Texture*:_____ [*RI*: moist = hydrated; tacky-to-dry = 5–12% dehydrated]

Physical Exam – Systems Checklist:

- Head:_____ ☐NAF
  - ◦ Ears: ☐Ceruminous debris (mild / mod / sev) (AS / AD / AU), _____ ☐NAF
  - ◦ Eyes:_____ ☐NAF
    - ▪ Retinal:_____ ☐NAF

→ ⓛ		ⓡ		ⓛ		ⓡ ←	
☐ ⊙ Normal Direct	☐ ⊙ Normal Indirect	☐ ⊙ Normal Indirect	☐ ⊙ Normal Direct
☐ ● Abnormal Direct	☐ ● Abnormal Indirect	☐ ● Abnormal Indirect	☐ ● Abnormal Direct

  - ◦ Nose:_____ ☐NAF
  - ◦ Oral cavity: ☐Tarter/Gingivitis (mild / mod / sev), _____ ☐NAF
  - ◦ Mandibular lnn.: ☐Enlarged Lt., ☐Enlarged Rt., _____ ☐NAF

- Neck:_____ ☐NAF
  - ◦ Superficial cervical lnn.: ☐Enlarged Lt., ☐Enlarged Rt., _____ ☐NAF
  - ◦ Thyroid:_____ ☐NAF

- Thoracic limb:_____ ☐NAF
  - ◦ Foot pads:_____ ☐NAF
  - ◦ Knuckling:_____ ☐NAF
  - ◦ Axillary lnn. [normally absent]:_____ ☐NAF

- Thorax:_____ ☐NAF

- Abdomen:_____ ☐NAF
  - ◦ Mammary chain:_____ ☐NAF
  - ◦ Penis/ Testicles/ Vulva:_____ ☐NAF
  - ◦ Superficial inguinal lnn. [normally absent]:_____ ☐NAF

- Pelvic limb:_____ ☐NAF
  - ◦ Foot pads:_____ ☐NAF
  - ◦ Knuckling:_____ ☐NAF
  - ◦ Popliteal lnn.: ☐Enlarged Lt., ☐Enlarged Rt., _____ ☐NAF

- Skin:_____ ☐NAF
- Tail:_____ ☐NAF
- Rectal☞☉:_____ ☐NAF

Problems List:

- **Problem #1**:

- **Problem #2**:

- **Problem #3**:

- **Problem #4**:

- **Problem #5**:

- **Problem #6**:

Diagnostic Plan	Treatment Plan

Case No._____

Patient	Age	Sex		Breed		Weight
		nM	sF			
	DOB:	iM	iF	Color:		kg

Owner	Primary Veterinarian	Admit Date/ Time
Name: Phone:	Name: Phone:	Date: Time: AM / PM

• **Presenting complaint**:_____
_____
_____
_____
_____
_____

• **Medical Hx**:_____
_____
_____
_____
_____

• **When/ where obtained**: Date:_____; ☐Breeder, ☐Shelter, Other:_____

Drug/ Supplement	Amount	Dose (mg/kg)	Route	Frequency	Date Started

• **Vaccine status – Dog**: ☐Rab ☐Parv ☐Dist ☐Aden; ☐Para ☐Lep ☐Bord ☐Influ ☐Lyme
• **Vaccine status – Cat**: ☐Rab ☐Herp ☐Cali ☐Pan ☐FeLV [kittens]; ☐FIV ☐Chlam ☐Bord
• **Heartworm / Flea & Tick / Intestinal Parasites**:
   ◦ *Last Heartworm Test*: Date:_____, ☐IDK; Test Results: ☐Pos, ☐Neg, ☐IDK
   ◦ *Monthly heartworm preventative*: ☐no ☐yes, Product:_____
   ◦ *Monthly flea & tick preventative*: ☐no ☐yes, Product:_____
   ◦ *Monthly dewormer*: ☐no ☐yes, Product:_____
• **Surgical Hx**: ☐Spay/Neuter; Date:_____; Other:_____
• **Environment**: ☐Indoor, ☐Outdoor, Time spent outdoors/ Other:_____
• **Housemates**: Dogs:_____ Cats:_____ Other:_____
• **Diet**: ☐Wet, ☐Dry; Brand/ Amt.:_____

Appetite	☐Normal, ☐↑, ☐↓
Weight	☐Normal, ☐↑, ☐↓; Past Wt.:_____ kg; Date:_____; Δ:_____
Thirst	☐Normal, ☐↑, ☐↓
Urination	☐Normal, ☐↑, ☐↓, ☐Blood, ☐Strain
Defecation	☐Normal, ☐↑, ☐↓, ☐Blood, ☐Strain, ☐Diarrhea, ☐Mucus
Discharge	☐No, ☐Yes; Onset/ Describe:
Cough/ Sneeze	☐No, ☐Yes; Onset/ Describe:
Vomit	☐No, ☐Yes; Onset/ Describe:
Respiration	☐Normal, ☐↑ Rate, ☐↑ Effort
Energy level	☐Normal, ☐Lethargic, ☐Exercise intolerance

• **Travel Hx**: ☐None, Other:_____
• **Exposure to**: ☐Standing water, ☐Wildlife, ☐Board/daycare, ☐Dog park, ☐Groomer, ☐Pet store
• **Adverse reactions to food/ meds**: ☐None, Other:_____
• **Can give oral meds**: ☐no ☐yes; Helpful Tricks:_____

Physical Exam – General:

- **Body Weight**:_____kg   **Body Condition Score**:___/9

- **Temperature**:_____°F [*Dog-RI*: 100.9–102.4; *Cat-RI*: 98.1–102.1]

- **Heart**:
  - *Rate*:_____beats/min [Dog-RI: 60–180; Cat-RI: 140–240 (in hospital)]
  - *Rhythm*: □Regular, □Irregular
  - *Sounds*: □None, □Split sound[S1 or S2], □Gallop[S3 or S4], □Murmur, □Muffled
    - *Grade*: □1–2[soft, only at PMI], □3–4[moderate, mild radiate], □5–6[loud, strong radiate, thrill]
    - *Timing*: □Systolic, □Diastolic, □Continuous
    - *PMI*:

	PMI	Over	Anatomic Boundaries
□	Lt. apex	Mitral valve	5th to 6th ICS at level of CCJ
□	Lt. base	Ao + Pul outflow	2nd to 4th ICS above the CCJ
□	Rt. midheart	Tricuspid valve	3rd to 5th ICS near the CCJ
□	Rt. sternal border	Right ventricle	5th to 7th ICS immediately dorsal to the sternum
□	Sternal (cat)	Sternum	In cats, determination of PMI offers very little clinical significance.

  - *Vertebral Heart Size*: Dog = 8.7–10.7; Cat = 6.9–8.1 (from cranial edge of T4)
  - *Innocent Murmur*: Grade 1-2, systolic, left base location, disappear by ~4 months of age, absent clinical signs

- **Pulses**:
  - *Pulse rate*:_____pulses/min
  - *Character*: □Sync, □Async; □Normokinetic, □Hyper-, □Hypo-, □Variable

- **Lungs**:
  - *Respiratory rate*:_____breaths/min [*RI*: 16–30]
  - *Depth/Effort*: □Norm, □Pant, □Deep, □Shallow, □↑ Insp. effort, □↑ Exp. effort
  - *Sounds/Localization*:
    - □Norm BV, □Quiet BV, □Loud BV, □Crack, □Wheez, □Frict, □Muffled
    - □All lung fields, □Rt cran, □Rt mid, □Rt caud, □Lt cran, □Lt mid, □Lt caud
  - *Tracheal Auscultation/ Palpation*: □Normal, Other:_____

- **Pain Score**:_____ / 5   Localization:_____

- **Mentation**: □BAR   □Confused/   □Drowsy/   □Stuporous   □Coma

  □QAR   Disoriented   Obtunded

  □Dull

(conscious; responds to sensory stimuli)	(conscious; inappropriate response to environment [ex., vocalization, head pressing])	(↓ interaction with environment; slow response to verbal stimuli)	(unresponsive unless aroused by noxious stimuli)	(complete unresponsiveness to any stimuli)

- **Skin Elasticity**: □Normal skin turgor, □↓ Skin turgor, □Skin tent, □Gelatinous

- **Mucus Membranes**:
  - *CRT*:_____ [*RI*: 1–2; <1 = compensated shock, sepsis, heat stroke; <2 = acute decompensated shock; >2 = late decompensated shock, decreased cardiac output, hypothermia]
  - *Color*:_____ [*RI*: pink; red = compensated shock, sepsis, heat stroke; pale/white = anemia, shock; blue = cyanosis; yellow = hepatic disease, extravascular hemolysis; brown = met-Hb]
  - *Texture*:_____ [*RI*: moist = hydrated; tacky-to-dry = 5–12% dehydrated]

Physical Exam – Systems Checklist:

- Head:_____ ☐NAF
  - Ears: ☐Ceruminous debris (mild / mod / sev) (AS / AD / AU),_____ ☐NAF
  - Eyes:_____ ☐NAF
    - Retinal:_____ ☐NAF

→ Ⓛ		Ⓡ		Ⓛ		Ⓡ ←	
☐ ⊙ Normal Direct	☐ ⊙ Normal Indirect	☐ ⊙ Normal Indirect	☐ ⊙ Normal Direct
☐ ⊙ Abnormal Direct	☐ ⊙ Abnormal Indirect	☐ ⊙ Abnormal Indirect	☐ ⊙ Abnormal Direct

  - Nose:_____ ☐NAF
  - Oral cavity: ☐Tarter/Gingivitis (mild / mod / sev),_____ ☐NAF
  - Mandibular lnn.: ☐Enlarged Lt., ☐Enlarged Rt.,_____ ☐NAF

- Neck:_____ ☐NAF
  - Superficial cervical lnn.: ☐Enlarged Lt., ☐Enlarged Rt.,_____ ☐NAF
  - Thyroid:_____ ☐NAF

- Thoracic limb:_____ ☐NAF
  - Foot pads:_____ ☐NAF
  - Knuckling:_____ ☐NAF
  - Axillary lnn. [normally absent]:_____ ☐NAF

- Thorax:_____ ☐NAF

- Abdomen:_____ ☐NAF
  - Mammary chain:_____ ☐NAF
  - Penis/ Testicles/ Vulva:_____ ☐NAF
  - Superficial inguinal lnn. [normally absent]:_____ ☐NAF

- Pelvic limb:_____ ☐NAF
  - Foot pads:_____ ☐NAF
  - Knuckling:_____ ☐NAF
  - Popliteal lnn.: ☐Enlarged Lt., ☐Enlarged Rt.,_____ ☐NAF

- Skin:_____ ☐NAF
- Tail:_____ ☐NAF
- Rectal☞⊙:_____ ☐NAF

Problems List:

- **Problem #1**:

- **Problem #2**:

- **Problem #3**:

- **Problem #4**:

- **Problem #5**:

- **Problem #6**:

Diagnostic Plan	Treatment Plan

Case No._____

Patient	Age	Sex		Breed		Weight
		nM	sF			
	DOB:	iM	iF	Color:		kg

Owner	Primary Veterinarian	Admit Date/ Time
Name: Phone:	Name: Phone:	Date: Time: AM / PM

• **Presenting complaint**:_____
_____
_____
_____
_____
_____

• **Medical Hx**:_____
_____
_____
_____
_____

• **When/ where obtained**: Date:_____; ☐Breeder, ☐Shelter, Other:_____

Drug/ Supplement	Amount	Dose (mg/kg)	Route	Frequency	Date Started

• **Vaccine status – Dog**: ☐Rab ☐Parv ☐Dist ☐Aden; ☐Para ☐Lep ☐Bord ☐Influ ☐Lyme
• **Vaccine status – Cat**: ☐Rab ☐Herp ☐Cali ☐Pan ☐FeLV [kittens]; ☐FIV ☐Chlam ☐Bord
• **Heartworm / Flea & Tick / Intestinal Parasites**:
  ◦ *Last Heartworm Test*: Date:_____, ☐IDK; Test Results: ☐Pos, ☐Neg, ☐IDK
  ◦ *Monthly heartworm preventative*: ☐no ☐yes, Product:_____
  ◦ *Monthly flea & tick preventative*: ☐no ☐yes, Product:_____
  ◦ *Monthly dewormer*: ☐no ☐yes, Product:_____
• **Surgical Hx**: ☐Spay/Neuter; Date:_____; Other:_____
• **Environment**: ☐Indoor, ☐Outdoor, Time spent outdoors/ Other:_____
• **Housemates**: Dogs:_____ Cats:_____ Other:_____
• **Diet**: ☐Wet, ☐Dry; Brand/ Amt.:_____

Appetite	☐Normal, ☐↑, ☐↓
Weight	☐Normal, ☐↑, ☐↓; Past Wt.:_____ kg; Date:_____; Δ:_____
Thirst	☐Normal, ☐↑, ☐↓
Urination	☐Normal, ☐↑, ☐↓, ☐Blood, ☐Strain
Defecation	☐Normal, ☐↑, ☐↓, ☐Blood, ☐Strain, ☐Diarrhea, ☐Mucus
Discharge	☐No, ☐Yes; Onset/ Describe:
Cough/ Sneeze	☐No, ☐Yes; Onset/ Describe:
Vomit	☐No, ☐Yes; Onset/ Describe:
Respiration	☐Normal, ☐↑ Rate, ☐↑ Effort
Energy level	☐Normal, ☐Lethargic, ☐Exercise intolerance

• **Travel Hx**: ☐None, Other:_____
• **Exposure to**: ☐Standing water, ☐Wildlife, ☐Board/daycare, ☐Dog park, ☐Groomer, ☐Pet store
• **Adverse reactions to food/ meds**: ☐None, Other:_____
• **Can give oral meds**: ☐no ☐yes; Helpful Tricks:_____

Physical Exam – General:

- **Body Weight**:_____kg   **Body Condition Score**:____/9

- **Temperature**:_____°F [*Dog-RI*: 100.9–102.4; *Cat-RI*: 98.1–102.1]

- **Heart**:
  - *Rate*:_____beats/min [Dog-RI: 60–180; Cat-RI: 140–240 (in hospital)]
  - *Rhythm*: ☐Regular, ☐Irregular
  - *Sounds*: ☐None, ☐Split sound[S1 or S2], ☐Gallop[S3 or S4], ☐Murmur, ☐Muffled
    - *Grade*: ☐1–2[soft, only at PMI], ☐3–4[moderate, mild radiate], ☐5–6[loud, strong radiate, thrill]
    - *Timing*: ☐Systolic, ☐Diastolic, ☐Continuous
    - *PMI*:

	PMI	Over	Anatomic Boundaries
☐	Lt. apex	Mitral valve	5th to 6th ICS at level of CCJ
☐	Lt. base	Ao + Pul outflow	2nd to 4th ICS above the CCJ
☐	Rt. midheart	Tricuspid valve	3rd to 5th ICS near the CCJ
☐	Rt. sternal border	Right ventricle	5th to 7th ICS immediately dorsal to the sternum
☐	Sternal (cat)	Sternum	In cats, determination of PMI offers very little clinical significance.

  - *Vertebral Heart Size*: Dog = 8.7–10.7; Cat = 6.9–8.1 (from cranial edge of T4)
  - *Innocent Murmur*: Grade 1-2, systolic, left base location, disappear by ~4 months of age, absent clinical signs

- **Pulses**:
  - *Pulse rate*:_____pulses/min
  - *Character*: ☐Sync, ☐Async; ☐Normokinetic, ☐Hyper-, ☐Hypo-, ☐Variable

- **Lungs**:
  - *Respiratory rate*:_____breaths/min [*RI*: 16–30]
  - *Depth/Effort*: ☐Norm, ☐Pant, ☐Deep, ☐Shallow, ☐↑ Insp. effort, ☐↑ Exp. effort
  - *Sounds/Localization*:
    - ☐Norm BV, ☐Quiet BV, ☐Loud BV, ☐Crack, ☐Wheez, ☐Frict, ☐Muffled
    - ☐All lung fields, ☐Rt cran, ☐Rt mid, ☐Rt caud, ☐Lt cran, ☐Lt mid, ☐Lt caud
  - *Tracheal Auscultation/ Palpation*: ☐Normal, Other:_____

- **Pain Score**:_____ / 5   Localization:_____

- **Mentation**:

☐BAR	☐Confused/	☐Drowsy/	☐Stuporous	☐Coma
☐QAR	Disoriented	Obtunded	(unresponsive unless aroused by noxious stimuli)	(complete unresponsiveness to any stimuli)
☐Dull (conscious; responds to sensory stimuli)	(conscious; inappropriate response to environment [ex., vocalization, head pressing])	(↓ interaction with environment; slow response to verbal stimuli)		

- **Skin Elasticity**: ☐Normal skin turgor, ☐↓ Skin turgor, ☐Skin tent, ☐Gelatinous

- **Mucus Membranes**:
  - *CRT*:_____ [*RI*: 1–2; <1 = compensated shock, sepsis, heat stroke; <2 = acute decompensated shock; >2 = late decompensated shock, decreased cardiac output, hypothermia]
  - *Color*:_____ [*RI*: pink; red = compensated shock, sepsis, heat stroke; pale/white = anemia, shock; blue = cyanosis; yellow = hepatic disease, extravascular hemolysis; brown = met-Hb]
  - *Texture*:_____ [*RI*: moist = hydrated; tacky-to-dry = 5–12% dehydrated]

Physical Exam – Systems Checklist:

- Head: _____ ☐NAF
  - Ears: ☐Ceruminous debris (mild / mod / sev) (AS / AD / AU), _____ ☐NAF
  - Eyes: _____ ☐NAF
    - Retinal: _____ ☐NAF

→ Ⓛ		Ⓡ		Ⓛ		Ⓡ ←	
☐	⊙ Normal Direct	☐	⊙ Normal Indirect	☐	⊙ Normal Indirect	☐	⊙ Normal Direct
☐	⊙ Abnormal Direct	☐	⊙ Abnormal Indirect	☐	⊙ Abnormal Indirect	☐	⊙ Abnormal Direct

  - Nose: _____ ☐NAF
  - Oral cavity: ☐Tarter/Gingivitis (mild / mod / sev), _____ ☐NAF
  - Mandibular lnn.: ☐Enlarged Lt., ☐Enlarged Rt., _____ ☐NAF

- Neck: _____ ☐NAF
  - Superficial cervical lnn.: ☐Enlarged Lt., ☐Enlarged Rt., _____ ☐NAF
  - Thyroid: _____ ☐NAF

- Thoracic limb: _____ ☐NAF
  - Foot pads: _____ ☐NAF
  - Knuckling: _____ ☐NAF
  - Axillary lnn. [normally absent]: _____ ☐NAF

- Thorax: _____ ☐NAF

- Abdomen: _____ ☐NAF
  - Mammary chain: _____ ☐NAF
  - Penis/ Testicles/ Vulva: _____ ☐NAF
  - Superficial inguinal lnn. [normally absent]: _____ ☐NAF

- Pelvic limb: _____ ☐NAF
  - Foot pads: _____ ☐NAF
  - Knuckling: _____ ☐NAF
  - Popliteal lnn.: ☐Enlarged Lt., ☐Enlarged Rt., _____ ☐NAF

- Skin: _____ ☐NAF
- Tail: _____ ☐NAF
- Rectal☞⊙: _____ ☐NAF

Problems List:

- **Problem #1**:

- **Problem #2**:

- **Problem #3**:

- **Problem #4**:

- **Problem #5**:

- **Problem #6**:

Diagnostic Plan	Treatment Plan

Case No._____

Patient	Age	Sex		Breed		Weight
		nM	sF			
	DOB:	iM	iF	Color:		kg

Owner	Primary Veterinarian	Admit Date/ Time
Name: Phone:	Name: Phone:	Date: Time: AM / PM

• **Presenting complaint**:_____
_____
_____
_____
_____
_____

• **Medical Hx**:_____
_____
_____
_____
_____

• **When/ where obtained**: Date:_____; ☐Breeder, ☐Shelter, Other:_____

Drug/ Supplement	Amount	Dose (mg/kg)	Route	Frequency	Date Started

• **Vaccine status – Dog**: ☐Rab ☐Parv ☐Dist ☐Aden; ☐Para ☐Lep ☐Bord ☐Influ ☐Lyme
• **Vaccine status – Cat**: ☐Rab ☐Herp ☐Cali ☐Pan ☐FeLV [kittens]; ☐FIV ☐Chlam ☐Bord
• **Heartworm / Flea & Tick / Intestinal Parasites**:
  ◦ *Last Heartworm Test*: Date:_____, ☐IDK; Test Results: ☐Pos, ☐Neg, ☐IDK
  ◦ *Monthly heartworm preventative*: ☐no ☐yes, Product:_____
  ◦ *Monthly flea & tick preventative*: ☐no ☐yes, Product:_____
  ◦ *Monthly dewormer*:   ☐no ☐yes, Product:_____
• **Surgical Hx**: ☐Spay/Neuter; Date:_____; Other:_____
• **Environment**: ☐Indoor, ☐Outdoor, Time spent outdoors/ Other:_____
• **Housemates**: Dogs:_____ Cats:_____ Other:_____
• **Diet**: ☐Wet, ☐Dry; Brand/ Amt.:_____

Appetite	☐Normal, ☐↑, ☐↓
Weight	☐Normal, ☐↑, ☐↓; Past Wt.:_____ kg; Date:_____; Δ:_____
Thirst	☐Normal, ☐↑, ☐↓
Urination	☐Normal, ☐↑, ☐↓, ☐Blood, ☐Strain
Defecation	☐Normal, ☐↑, ☐↓, ☐Blood, ☐Strain, ☐Diarrhea, ☐Mucus
Discharge	☐No, ☐Yes; Onset/ Describe:
Cough/ Sneeze	☐No, ☐Yes; Onset/ Describe:
Vomit	☐No, ☐Yes; Onset/ Describe:
Respiration	☐Normal, ☐↑ Rate, ☐↑ Effort
Energy level	☐Normal, ☐Lethargic, ☐Exercise intolerance

• **Travel Hx**: ☐None, Other:_____
• **Exposure to**: ☐Standing water, ☐Wildlife, ☐Board/daycare, ☐Dog park, ☐Groomer, ☐Pet store
• **Adverse reactions to food/ meds**: ☐None, Other:_____
• **Can give oral meds**: ☐no ☐yes; Helpful Tricks:_____

Physical Exam – General:

- **Body Weight:**_____kg   **Body Condition Score:**___/9

- **Temperature:**_____°F [*Dog-RI*: 100.9–102.4; *Cat-RI*: 98.1–102.1]

- **Heart:**
  - *Rate*:_____beats/min [Dog-RI: 60–180; Cat-RI: 140–240 (in hospital)]
  - *Rhythm*: ☐Regular, ☐Irregular
  - *Sounds*: ☐None, ☐Split sound[S1 or S2], ☐Gallop[S3 or S4], ☐Murmur, ☐Muffled
    - *Grade*: ☐1–2[soft, only at PMI], ☐3–4[moderate, mild radiate], ☐5–6[loud, strong radiate, thrill]
    - *Timing*: ☐Systolic, ☐Diastolic, ☐Continuous
    - *PMI*:

	PMI	Over	Anatomic Boundaries
☐	Lt. apex	Mitral valve	5th to 6th ICS at level of CCJ
☐	Lt. base	Ao + Pul outflow	2nd to 4th ICS above the CCJ
☐	Rt. midheart	Tricuspid valve	3rd to 5th ICS near the CCJ
☐	Rt. sternal border	Right ventricle	5th to 7th ICS immediately dorsal to the sternum
☐	Sternal (cat)	Sternum	In cats, determination of PMI offers very little clinical significance.

  - • *Vertebral Heart Size*: Dog = 8.7–10.7; Cat = 6.9–8.1 (from cranial edge of T4)
  - • *Innocent Murmur*: Grade 1-2, systolic, left base location, disappear by ~4 months of age, absent clinical signs

- **Pulses:**
  - *Pulse rate*:_____pulses/min
  - *Character*: ☐Sync, ☐Async; ☐Normokinetic, ☐Hyper-, ☐Hypo-, ☐Variable

- **Lungs:**
  - *Respiratory rate*:_____breaths/min [*RI*: 16–30]
  - *Depth/Effort*: ☐Norm, ☐Pant, ☐Deep, ☐Shallow, ☐↑ Insp. effort, ☐↑ Exp. effort
  - *Sounds/Localization*:
    - ☐Norm BV, ☐Quiet BV, ☐Loud BV, ☐Crack, ☐Wheez, ☐Frict, ☐Muffled
    - ☐All lung fields, ☐Rt cran, ☐Rt mid, ☐Rt caud, ☐Lt cran, ☐Lt mid, ☐Lt caud
  - *Tracheal Auscultation/ Palpation*: ☐Normal, Other:_____

- **Pain Score:**_____ / 5   Localization:_____

- **Mentation**: ☐BAR   ☐Confused/   ☐Drowsy/   ☐Stuporous   ☐Coma
  ☐QAR   Disoriented   Obtunded   (unresponsive unless   (complete
  ☐Dull   (conscious; inappropriate   (↓ interaction with   aroused by noxious   unresponsiveness
  (conscious; responds   response to environment   environment; slow   stimuli)   to any stimuli)
  to sensory stimuli)   [ex., vocalization, head   response to verbal
  pressing])   stimuli)

- **Skin Elasticity**: ☐Normal skin turgor, ☐↓ Skin turgor, ☐Skin tent, ☐Gelatinous

- **Mucus Membranes:**
  - *CRT*:_____ [*RI*: 1–2; <1 = compensated shock, sepsis, heat stroke; <2 = acute decompensated shock;
    >2 = late decompensated shock, decreased cardiac output, hypothermia]
  - *Color*:_____ [*RI*: pink; red = compensated shock, sepsis, heat stroke; pale/white = anemia, shock;
    blue = cyanosis; yellow = hepatic disease, extravascular hemolysis; brown = met-Hb]
  - *Texture*:_____ [*RI*: moist = hydrated; tacky-to-dry = 5–12% dehydrated]

Physical Exam – Systems Checklist:

- Head: _____ ☐NAF
  - ○ Ears: ☐Ceruminous debris (mild / mod / sev) (AS / AD / AU), _____ ☐NAF
  - ○ Eyes: _____ ☐NAF
    - ▪ Retinal: _____ ☐NAF

→ Ⓛ		Ⓡ		Ⓛ		Ⓡ ←	
☐	⦿ Normal Direct	☐	⦿ Normal Indirect	☐	⦿ Normal Indirect	☐	⦿ Normal Direct
☐	⦿ Abnormal Direct	☐	● Abnormal Indirect	☐	● Abnormal Indirect	☐	⦿ Abnormal Direct

  - ○ Nose: _____ ☐NAF
  - ○ Oral cavity: ☐Tarter/Gingivitis (mild / mod / sev), _____ ☐NAF
  - ○ Mandibular lnn.: ☐Enlarged Lt., ☐Enlarged Rt., _____ ☐NAF

- Neck: _____ ☐NAF
  - ○ Superficial cervical lnn.: ☐Enlarged Lt., ☐Enlarged Rt., _____ ☐NAF
  - ○ Thyroid: _____ ☐NAF

- Thoracic limb: _____ ☐NAF
  - ○ Foot pads: _____ ☐NAF
  - ○ Knuckling: _____ ☐NAF
  - ○ Axillary lnn. [normally absent]: _____ ☐NAF

- Thorax: _____ ☐NAF

- Abdomen: _____ ☐NAF
  - ○ Mammary chain: _____ ☐NAF
  - ○ Penis/ Testicles/ Vulva: _____ ☐NAF
  - ○ Superficial inguinal lnn. [normally absent]: _____ ☐NAF

- Pelvic limb: _____ ☐NAF
  - ○ Foot pads: _____ ☐NAF
  - ○ Knuckling: _____ ☐NAF
  - ○ Popliteal lnn.: ☐Enlarged Lt., ☐Enlarged Rt., _____ ☐NAF

- Skin: _____ ☐NAF
- Tail: _____ ☐NAF
- Rectal☞☉: _____ ☐NAF

Problems List:

- **Problem #1**:

- **Problem #2**:

- **Problem #3**:

- **Problem #4**:

- **Problem #5**:

- **Problem #6**:

Diagnostic Plan	Treatment Plan

Case No._____

Patient	Age	Sex		Breed		Weight
		nM	sF			
	DOB:	iM	iF	Color:		kg

Owner	Primary Veterinarian	Admit Date/ Time
Name: Phone:	Name: Phone:	Date: Time: AM / PM

• **Presenting complaint**:_____
_____
_____
_____
_____
_____

• **Medical Hx**:_____
_____
_____
_____
_____

• **When/ where obtained**: Date:_____; ☐Breeder, ☐Shelter, Other:_____

Drug/ Supplement	Amount	Dose (mg/kg)	Route	Frequency	Date Started

• **Vaccine status – Dog**: ☐Rab ☐Parv ☐Dist ☐Aden; ☐Para ☐Lep ☐Bord ☐Influ ☐Lyme
• **Vaccine status – Cat**: ☐Rab ☐Herp ☐Cali ☐Pan ☐FeLV [kittens]; ☐FIV ☐Chlam ☐Bord
• **Heartworm / Flea & Tick / Intestinal Parasites**:
   ◦ *Last Heartworm Test*: Date:_____, ☐IDK; Test Results: ☐Pos, ☐Neg, ☐IDK
   ◦ *Monthly heartworm preventative*: ☐no ☐yes, Product:_____
   ◦ *Monthly flea & tick preventative*: ☐no ☐yes, Product:_____
   ◦ *Monthly dewormer*:   ☐no ☐yes, Product:_____
• **Surgical Hx**: ☐Spay/Neuter; Date:_____; Other:_____
• **Environment**: ☐Indoor, ☐Outdoor, Time spent outdoors/ Other:_____
• **Housemates**: Dogs:_____ Cats:_____ Other:_____
• **Diet**: ☐Wet, ☐Dry; Brand/ Amt.:_____

Appetite	☐Normal, ☐↑, ☐↓
Weight	☐Normal, ☐↑, ☐↓; Past Wt.:_____ kg; Date:_____; Δ:_____
Thirst	☐Normal, ☐↑, ☐↓
Urination	☐Normal, ☐↑, ☐↓, ☐Blood, ☐Strain
Defecation	☐Normal, ☐↑, ☐↓, ☐Blood, ☐Strain, ☐Diarrhea, ☐Mucus
Discharge	☐No, ☐Yes; Onset/ Describe:
Cough/ Sneeze	☐No, ☐Yes; Onset/ Describe:
Vomit	☐No, ☐Yes; Onset/ Describe:
Respiration	☐Normal, ☐↑ Rate, ☐↑ Effort
Energy level	☐Normal, ☐Lethargic, ☐Exercise intolerance

• **Travel Hx**: ☐None, Other:_____
• **Exposure to**: ☐Standing water, ☐Wildlife, ☐Board/daycare, ☐Dog park, ☐Groomer, ☐Pet store
• **Adverse reactions to food/ meds**: ☐None, Other:_____
• **Can give oral meds**: ☐no ☐yes; Helpful Tricks:_____

Physical Exam – General:

- **Body Weight:**_____kg   **Body Condition Score:**___/9

- **Temperature:**_____°F [*Dog-RI*: 100.9–102.4; *Cat-RI*: 98.1–102.1]

- **Heart:**
  - *Rate*:_____beats/min [Dog-RI: 60–180; Cat-RI: 140–240 (in hospital)]
  - *Rhythm*: □Regular, □Irregular
  - *Sounds*: □None, □Split sound[S1 or S2], □Gallop[S3 or S4], □Murmur, □Muffled
    - *Grade*: □1–2[soft, only at PMI], □3–4[moderate, mild radiate], □5–6[loud, strong radiate, thrill]
    - *Timing*: □Systolic, □Diastolic, □Continuous
    - *PMI*:

	PMI	Over	Anatomic Boundaries
□	Lt. apex	Mitral valve	5th to 6th ICS at level of CCJ
□	Lt. base	Ao + Pul outflow	2nd to 4th ICS above the CCJ
□	Rt. midheart	Tricuspid valve	3rd to 5th ICS near the CCJ
□	Rt. sternal border	Right ventricle	5th to 7th ICS immediately dorsal to the sternum
□	Sternal (cat)	Sternum	In cats, determination of PMI offers very little clinical significance.

    - *Vertebral Heart Size*: Dog = 8.7–10.7; Cat = 6.9–8.1 (from cranial edge of T4)
    - *Innocent Murmur*: Grade 1-2, systolic, left base location, disappear by ~4 months of age, absent clinical signs

- **Pulses:**
  - *Pulse rate*:_____pulses/min
  - *Character*: □Sync, □Async; □Normokinetic, □Hyper-, □Hypo-, □Variable

- **Lungs:**
  - *Respiratory rate*:_____breaths/min [*RI*: 16–30]
  - *Depth/Effort*: □Norm, □Pant, □Deep, □Shallow, □↑ Insp. effort, □↑ Exp. effort
  - *Sounds/Localization*:
    - □Norm BV, □Quiet BV, □Loud BV, □Crack, □Wheez, □Frict, □Muffled
    - □All lung fields, □Rt cran, □Rt mid, □Rt caud, □Lt cran, □Lt mid, □Lt caud
  - *Tracheal Auscultation/ Palpation*: □Normal, Other:_____

- **Pain Score:**_____ / 5   Localization:_____

- **Mentation**:

□BAR □QAR □Dull (conscious; responds to sensory stimuli)	□Confused/ Disoriented (conscious; inappropriate response to environment [ex., vocalization, head pressing])	□Drowsy/ Obtunded (↓ interaction with environment; slow response to verbal stimuli)	□Stuporous (unresponsive unless aroused by noxious stimuli)	□Coma (complete unresponsiveness to any stimuli)

- **Skin Elasticity**: □Normal skin turgor, □↓ Skin turgor, □Skin tent, □Gelatinous

- **Mucus Membranes:**
  - *CRT*:_____ [*RI*: 1–2; <1 = compensated shock, sepsis, heat stroke; <2 = acute decompensated shock; >2 = late decompensated shock, decreased cardiac output, hypothermia]
  - *Color*:_____ [*RI*: pink; red = compensated shock, sepsis, heat stroke; pale/white = anemia, shock; blue = cyanosis; yellow = hepatic disease, extravascular hemolysis; brown = met-Hb]
  - *Texture*:_____ [*RI*: moist = hydrated; tacky-to-dry = 5–12% dehydrated]

Physical Exam – Systems Checklist:

- Head: _____ ☐NAF
    - ◦ Ears: ☐Ceruminous debris (mild / mod / sev) (AS / AD / AU), _____ ☐NAF
    - ◦ Eyes: _____ ☐NAF
        - ▪ Retinal: _____ ☐NAF

→ Ⓛ		Ⓡ		Ⓛ		Ⓡ ←	
☐ ⊙ Normal Direct		☐ ⊙ Normal Indirect		☐ ⊙ Normal Indirect		☐ ⊙ Normal Direct	
☐ ⬤ Abnormal Direct		☐ ⬤ Abnormal Indirect		☐ ⬤ Abnormal Indirect		☐ ⬤ Abnormal Direct	

-
    - ◦ Nose: _____ ☐NAF
    - ◦ Oral cavity: ☐Tarter/Gingivitis (mild / mod / sev), _____ ☐NAF
    - ◦ Mandibular lnn.: ☐Enlarged Lt., ☐Enlarged Rt., _____ ☐NAF

- Neck: _____ ☐NAF
    - ◦ Superficial cervical lnn.: ☐Enlarged Lt., ☐Enlarged Rt., _____ ☐NAF
    - ◦ Thyroid: _____ ☐NAF

- Thoracic limb: _____ ☐NAF
    - ◦ Foot pads: _____ ☐NAF
    - ◦ Knuckling: _____ ☐NAF
    - ◦ Axillary lnn. [normally absent]: _____ ☐NAF

- Thorax: _____ ☐NAF

- Abdomen: _____ ☐NAF
    - ◦ Mammary chain: _____ ☐NAF
    - ◦ Penis/ Testicles/ Vulva: _____ ☐NAF
    - ◦ Superficial inguinal lnn. [normally absent]: _____ ☐NAF

- Pelvic limb: _____ ☐NAF
    - ◦ Foot pads: _____ ☐NAF
    - ◦ Knuckling: _____ ☐NAF
    - ◦ Popliteal lnn.: ☐Enlarged Lt., ☐Enlarged Rt., _____ ☐NAF

- Skin: _____ ☐NAF
- Tail: _____ ☐NAF
- Rectal ☞ ☉: _____ ☐NAF

Problems List:

• **Problem #1**:

• **Problem #2**:

• **Problem #3**:

• **Problem #4**:

• **Problem #5**:

• **Problem #6**:

Diagnostic Plan	Treatment Plan

Case No._____

Patient	Age	Sex		Breed	Weight
		nM	sF		
	DOB:	iM	iF	Color:	kg

Owner	Primary Veterinarian	Admit Date/ Time
Name: Phone:	Name: Phone:	Date: Time: AM / PM

• **Presenting complaint**:_____
_____
_____
_____
_____
_____

• **Medical Hx**:_____
_____
_____
_____
_____

• **When/ where obtained**: Date:_____; ☐Breeder, ☐Shelter, Other:_____

Drug/ Supplement	Amount	Dose (mg/kg)	Route	Frequency	Date Started

• **Vaccine status – Dog**: ☐Rab ☐Parv ☐Dist ☐Aden; ☐Para ☐Lep ☐Bord ☐Influ ☐Lyme
• **Vaccine status – Cat**: ☐Rab ☐Herp ☐Cali ☐Pan ☐FeLV [kittens]; ☐FIV ☐Chlam ☐Bord
• **Heartworm / Flea & Tick / Intestinal Parasites**:
  ◦ *Last Heartworm Test*: Date:_____, ☐IDK; Test Results: ☐Pos, ☐Neg, ☐IDK
  ◦ *Monthly heartworm preventative*: ☐no ☐yes, Product:_____
  ◦ *Monthly flea & tick preventative*: ☐no ☐yes, Product:_____
  ◦ *Monthly dewormer*:   ☐no ☐yes, Product:_____
• **Surgical Hx**: ☐Spay/Neuter; Date:_____; Other:_____
• **Environment**: ☐Indoor, ☐Outdoor, Time spent outdoors/ Other:_____
• **Housemates**: Dogs:_____ Cats:_____ Other:_____
• **Diet**: ☐Wet, ☐Dry; Brand/ Amt.:_____

Appetite	☐Normal, ☐↑, ☐↓
Weight	☐Normal, ☐↑, ☐↓; Past Wt.:_____ kg; Date:_____; Δ:_____
Thirst	☐Normal, ☐↑, ☐↓
Urination	☐Normal, ☐↑, ☐↓, ☐Blood, ☐Strain
Defecation	☐Normal, ☐↑, ☐↓, ☐Blood, ☐Strain, ☐Diarrhea, ☐Mucus
Discharge	☐No, ☐Yes; Onset/ Describe:
Cough/ Sneeze	☐No, ☐Yes; Onset/ Describe:
Vomit	☐No, ☐Yes; Onset/ Describe:
Respiration	☐Normal, ☐↑ Rate, ☐↑ Effort
Energy level	☐Normal, ☐Lethargic, ☐Exercise intolerance

• **Travel Hx**: ☐None, Other:_____
• **Exposure to**: ☐Standing water, ☐Wildlife, ☐Board/daycare, ☐Dog park, ☐Groomer, ☐Pet store
• **Adverse reactions to food/ meds**: ☐None, Other:_____
• **Can give oral meds**: ☐no ☐yes; Helpful Tricks:_____

Physical Exam – General:

- **Body Weight:**_____kg   **Body Condition Score:**____/9

- **Temperature:**_____°F [*Dog-RI*: 100.9–102.4; *Cat-RI*: 98.1–102.1]

- **Heart:**
  - *Rate*:_____beats/min [Dog-RI: 60–180; Cat-RI: 140–240 (in hospital)]
  - *Rhythm*: ☐Regular, ☐Irregular
  - *Sounds*: ☐None, ☐Split sound[S1 or S2], ☐Gallop[S3 or S4], ☐Murmur, ☐Muffled
    - *Grade*: ☐1–2[soft, only at PMI], ☐3–4[moderate, mild radiate], ☐5–6[loud, strong radiate, thrill]
    - *Timing*: ☐Systolic, ☐Diastolic, ☐Continuous
    - *PMI*:

	PMI	Over	Anatomic Boundaries
☐	Lt. apex	Mitral valve	5th to 6th ICS at level of CCJ
☐	Lt. base	Ao + Pul outflow	2nd to 4th ICS above the CCJ
☐	Rt. midheart	Tricuspid valve	3rd to 5th ICS near the CCJ
☐	Rt. sternal border	Right ventricle	5th to 7th ICS immediately dorsal to the sternum
☐	Sternal (cat)	Sternum	In cats, determination of PMI offers very little clinical significance.

  - • *Vertebral Heart Size*: Dog = 8.7–10.7; Cat = 6.9–8.1 (from cranial edge of T4)
  - • *Innocent Murmur*: Grade 1-2, systolic, left base location, disappear by ~4 months of age, absent clinical signs

- **Pulses:**
  - *Pulse rate*:_____pulses/min
  - *Character*: ☐Sync, ☐Async; ☐Normokinetic, ☐Hyper-, ☐Hypo-, ☐Variable

- **Lungs:**
  - *Respiratory rate*:_____breaths/min [*RI*: 16–30]
  - *Depth/Effort*: ☐Norm, ☐Pant, ☐Deep, ☐Shallow, ☐↑ Insp. effort, ☐↑ Exp. effort
  - *Sounds/Localization*:
    - ☐Norm BV, ☐Quiet BV, ☐Loud BV, ☐Crack, ☐Wheez, ☐Frict, ☐Muffled
    - ☐All lung fields, ☐Rt cran, ☐Rt mid, ☐Rt caud, ☐Lt cran, ☐Lt mid, ☐Lt caud
  - *Tracheal Auscultation/ Palpation*: ☐Normal, Other:_____

- **Pain Score:**_____ / 5   Localization:_____

- **Mentation:** ☐BAR ☐Confused/ ☐Drowsy/ ☐Stuporous ☐Coma
  - ☐QAR Disoriented Obtunded (unresponsive unless (complete
  - ☐Dull (conscious; inappropriate (↓ interaction with aroused by noxious unresponsiveness
  - (conscious; responds response to environment environment; slow stimuli) to any stimuli)
  - to sensory stimuli) [ex., vocalization, head response to verbal
  - pressing]) stimuli)

- **Skin Elasticity:** ☐Normal skin turgor, ☐↓ Skin turgor, ☐Skin tent, ☐Gelatinous

- **Mucus Membranes:**
  - *CRT*:_____ [*RI*: 1–2; <1 = compensated shock, sepsis, heat stroke; <2 = acute decompensated shock; >2 = late decompensated shock, decreased cardiac output, hypothermia]
  - *Color*:_____ [*RI*: pink; red = compensated shock, sepsis, heat stroke; pale/white = anemia, shock; blue = cyanosis; yellow = hepatic disease, extravascular hemolysis; brown = met-Hb]
  - *Texture*:_____ [*RI*: moist = hydrated; tacky-to-dry = 5–12% dehydrated]

Physical Exam – Systems Checklist:

- Head: _____ ☐NAF
  - Ears: ☐Ceruminous debris (mild / mod / sev) (AS / AD / AU), _____ ☐NAF
  - Eyes: _____ ☐NAF
    - Retinal: _____ ☐NAF

→ Ⓛ	Ⓡ	Ⓛ	Ⓡ ←
☐ ◉ Normal Direct	☐ ◉ Normal Indirect	☐ ◉ Normal Indirect	☐ ◉ Normal Direct
☐ ◉ Abnormal Direct	☐ ● Abnormal Indirect	☐ ● Abnormal Indirect	☐ ◉ Abnormal Direct

  - Nose: _____ ☐NAF
  - Oral cavity: ☐Tarter/Gingivitis (mild / mod / sev), _____ ☐NAF
  - Mandibular lnn.: ☐Enlarged Lt., ☐Enlarged Rt., _____ ☐NAF

- Neck: _____ ☐NAF
  - Superficial cervical lnn.: ☐Enlarged Lt., ☐Enlarged Rt., _____ ☐NAF
  - Thyroid: _____ ☐NAF

- Thoracic limb: _____ ☐NAF
  - Foot pads: _____ ☐NAF
  - Knuckling: _____ ☐NAF
  - Axillary lnn. [normally absent]: _____ ☐NAF

- Thorax: _____ ☐NAF

- Abdomen: _____ ☐NAF
  - Mammary chain: _____ ☐NAF
  - Penis/ Testicles/ Vulva: _____ ☐NAF
  - Superficial inguinal lnn. [normally absent]: _____ ☐NAF

- Pelvic limb: _____ ☐NAF
  - Foot pads: _____ ☐NAF
  - Knuckling: _____ ☐NAF
  - Popliteal lnn.: ☐Enlarged Lt., ☐Enlarged Rt., _____ ☐NAF

- Skin: _____ ☐NAF
- Tail: _____ ☐NAF
- Rectal ☞⊙: _____ ☐NAF

Problems List:

- **Problem #1**:

- **Problem #2**:

- **Problem #3**:

- **Problem #4**:

- **Problem #5**:

- **Problem #6**:

Diagnostic Plan	Treatment Plan

Case No._____

Patient	Age	Sex		Breed	Weight
		nM	sF		kg
	DOB:	iM	iF	Color:	

Owner	Primary Veterinarian	Admit Date/ Time
Name: Phone:	Name: Phone:	Date: Time: AM / PM

- **Presenting complaint**:_____
_____
_____
_____
_____

- **Medical Hx**:_____
_____
_____
_____
_____

- **When/ where obtained**: Date:_____; ☐Breeder, ☐Shelter, Other:_____

Drug/ Supplement	Amount	Dose (mg/kg)	Route	Frequency	Date Started

- **Vaccine status – Dog**: ☐Rab ☐Parv ☐Dist ☐Aden; ☐Para ☐Lep ☐Bord ☐Influ ☐Lyme
- **Vaccine status – Cat**: ☐Rab ☐Herp ☐Cali ☐Pan ☐FeLV [kittens]; ☐FIV ☐Chlam ☐Bord
- **Heartworm / Flea & Tick / Intestinal Parasites**:
  - *Last Heartworm Test*: Date:_____, ☐IDK; Test Results: ☐Pos, ☐Neg, ☐IDK
  - *Monthly heartworm preventative*: ☐no ☐yes, Product:_____
  - *Monthly flea & tick preventative*: ☐no ☐yes, Product:_____
  - *Monthly dewormer*:   ☐no ☐yes, Product:_____
- **Surgical Hx**: ☐Spay/Neuter; Date:_____; Other:_____
- **Environment**: ☐Indoor, ☐Outdoor, Time spent outdoors/ Other:_____
- **Housemates**: Dogs:_____ Cats:_____ Other:_____
- **Diet**: ☐Wet, ☐Dry; Brand/ Amt.:_____

Appetite	☐Normal, ☐↑, ☐↓
Weight	☐Normal, ☐↑, ☐↓; Past Wt.:_____ kg; Date:_____; Δ:_____
Thirst	☐Normal, ☐↑, ☐↓
Urination	☐Normal, ☐↑, ☐↓, ☐Blood, ☐Strain
Defecation	☐Normal, ☐↑, ☐↓, ☐Blood, ☐Strain, ☐Diarrhea, ☐Mucus
Discharge	☐No, ☐Yes; Onset/ Describe:
Cough/ Sneeze	☐No, ☐Yes; Onset/ Describe:
Vomit	☐No, ☐Yes; Onset/ Describe:
Respiration	☐Normal, ☐↑ Rate, ☐↑ Effort
Energy level	☐Normal, ☐Lethargic, ☐Exercise intolerance

- **Travel Hx**: ☐None, Other:_____
- **Exposure to**: ☐Standing water, ☐Wildlife, ☐Board/daycare, ☐Dog park, ☐Groomer, ☐Pet store
- **Adverse reactions to food/ meds**: ☐None, Other:_____
- **Can give oral meds**: ☐no ☐yes; Helpful Tricks:_____

Physical Exam – General:

- **Body Weight**:_____kg   **Body Condition Score**:___/9

- **Temperature**:_____°F [*Dog-RI*: 100.9–102.4; *Cat-RI*: 98.1–102.1]

- **Heart**:
  - *Rate*:_____beats/min [Dog-RI: 60–180; Cat-RI: 140–240 (in hospital)]
  - *Rhythm*: ☐Regular, ☐Irregular
  - *Sounds*: ☐None, ☐Split sound[S1 or S2], ☐Gallop[S3 or S4], ☐Murmur, ☐Muffled
    - *Grade*: ☐1–2[soft, only at PMI], ☐3–4[moderate, mild radiate], ☐5–6[loud, strong radiate, thrill]
    - *Timing*: ☐Systolic, ☐Diastolic, ☐Continuous
    - *PMI*:

	PMI	Over	Anatomic Boundaries
☐	Lt. apex	Mitral valve	5th to 6th ICS at level of CCJ
☐	Lt. base	Ao + Pul outflow	2nd to 4th ICS above the CCJ
☐	Rt. midheart	Tricuspid valve	3rd to 5th ICS near the CCJ
☐	Rt. sternal border	Right ventricle	5th to 7th ICS immediately dorsal to the sternum
☐	Sternal (cat)	Sternum	In cats, determination of PMI offers very little clinical significance.

  - *Vertebral Heart Size*: Dog = 8.7–10.7; Cat = 6.9–8.1 (from cranial edge of T4)
  - *Innocent Murmur*: Grade 1-2, systolic, left base location, disappear by ~4 months of age, absent clinical signs

- **Pulses**:
  - *Pulse rate*:_____pulses/min
  - *Character*: ☐Sync, ☐Async; ☐Normokinetic, ☐Hyper-, ☐Hypo-, ☐Variable

- **Lungs**:
  - *Respiratory rate*:_____breaths/min [*RI*: 16–30]
  - *Depth/Effort*: ☐Norm, ☐Pant, ☐Deep, ☐Shallow, ☐↑ Insp. effort, ☐↑ Exp. effort
  - *Sounds/Localization*:
    - ☐Norm BV, ☐Quiet BV, ☐Loud BV, ☐Crack, ☐Wheez, ☐Frict, ☐Muffled
    - ☐All lung fields, ☐Rt cran, ☐Rt mid, ☐Rt caud, ☐Lt cran, ☐Lt mid, ☐Lt caud
  - *Tracheal Auscultation/ Palpation*: ☐Normal, Other:_____

- **Pain Score**:_____ / 5   Localization:_____

- **Mentation**:

☐BAR ☐QAR ☐Dull (conscious; responds to sensory stimuli)	☐Confused/ Disoriented (conscious; inappropriate response to environment [ex., vocalization, head pressing])	☐Drowsy/ Obtunded (↓ interaction with environment; slow response to verbal stimuli)	☐Stuporous (unresponsive unless aroused by noxious stimuli)	☐Coma (complete unresponsiveness to any stimuli)

- **Skin Elasticity**: ☐Normal skin turgor, ☐↓ Skin turgor, ☐Skin tent, ☐Gelatinous

- **Mucus Membranes**:
  - *CRT*:_____[*RI*: 1–2; <1 = compensated shock, sepsis, heat stroke; <2 = acute decompensated shock; >2 = late decompensated shock, decreased cardiac output, hypothermia]
  - *Color*:_____[*RI*: pink; red = compensated shock, sepsis, heat stroke; pale/white = anemia, shock; blue = cyanosis; yellow = hepatic disease, extravascular hemolysis; brown = met-Hb]
  - *Texture*:_____[*RI*: moist = hydrated; tacky-to-dry = 5–12% dehydrated]

Physical Exam – Systems Checklist:

- **Head:** _____ ☐NAF
  - ○ Ears: ☐Ceruminous debris (mild / mod / sev) (AS / AD / AU), _____ ☐NAF
  - ○ Eyes: _____ ☐NAF
    - ▪ Retinal: _____ ☐NAF

→ ⓛ		ⓡ		ⓛ		ⓡ ←	
☐ ⊙ Normal Direct	☐ ⊙ Normal Indirect	☐ ⊙ Normal Indirect	☐ ⊙ Normal Direct
☐ ⊙ Abnormal Direct	☐ ⊙ Abnormal Indirect	☐ ⊙ Abnormal Indirect	☐ ⊙ Abnormal Direct

  - ○ Nose: _____ ☐NAF
  - ○ Oral cavity: ☐Tarter/Gingivitis (mild / mod / sev), _____ ☐NAF
  - ○ Mandibular lnn.: ☐Enlarged Lt., ☐Enlarged Rt., _____ ☐NAF

- **Neck:** _____ ☐NAF
  - ○ Superficial cervical lnn.: ☐Enlarged Lt., ☐Enlarged Rt., _____ ☐NAF
  - ○ Thyroid: _____ ☐NAF

- **Thoracic limb:** _____ ☐NAF
  - ○ Foot pads: _____ ☐NAF
  - ○ Knuckling: _____ ☐NAF
  - ○ Axillary lnn. [normally absent]: _____ ☐NAF

- **Thorax:** _____ ☐NAF

- **Abdomen:** _____ ☐NAF
  - ○ Mammary chain: _____ ☐NAF
  - ○ Penis/ Testicles/ Vulva: _____ ☐NAF
  - ○ Superficial inguinal lnn. [normally absent]: _____ ☐NAF

- **Pelvic limb:** _____ ☐NAF
  - ○ Foot pads: _____ ☐NAF
  - ○ Knuckling: _____ ☐NAF
  - ○ Popliteal lnn.: ☐Enlarged Lt., ☐Enlarged Rt., _____ ☐NAF

- **Skin:** _____ ☐NAF
- **Tail:** _____ ☐NAF
- **Rectal☞⊙:** _____ ☐NAF

118

Problems List:

• **Problem #1**:

• **Problem #2**:

• **Problem #3**:

• **Problem #4**:

• **Problem #5**:

• **Problem #6**:

Diagnostic Plan	Treatment Plan

Case No._____

Patient	Age	Sex		Breed	Weight
		nM	sF		
	DOB:	iM	iF	Color:	kg

Owner	Primary Veterinarian	Admit Date/ Time
Name: Phone:	Name: Phone:	Date: Time: AM / PM

• **Presenting complaint**:_____
_____
_____
_____
_____
_____

• **Medical Hx**:_____
_____
_____
_____
_____

• **When/ where obtained**: Date:_____; ☐Breeder, ☐Shelter, Other:_____

Drug/ Supplement	Amount	Dose (mg/kg)	Route	Frequency	Date Started

• **Vaccine status – Dog**: ☐Rab ☐Parv ☐Dist ☐Aden; ☐Para ☐Lep ☐Bord ☐Influ ☐Lyme
• **Vaccine status – Cat**: ☐Rab ☐Herp ☐Cali ☐Pan ☐FeLV [kittens]; ☐FIV ☐Chlam ☐Bord
• **Heartworm / Flea & Tick / Intestinal Parasites**:
  ◦ *Last Heartworm Test*: Date:_____, ☐IDK; Test Results: ☐Pos, ☐Neg, ☐IDK
  ◦ *Monthly heartworm preventative*: ☐no ☐yes, Product:_____
  ◦ *Monthly flea & tick preventative*: ☐no ☐yes, Product:_____
  ◦ *Monthly dewormer*: ☐no ☐yes, Product:_____
• **Surgical Hx**: ☐Spay/Neuter; Date:_____; Other:_____
• **Environment**: ☐Indoor, ☐Outdoor, Time spent outdoors/ Other:_____
• **Housemates**: Dogs:_____ Cats:_____ Other:_____
• **Diet**: ☐Wet, ☐Dry; Brand/ Amt.:_____

Appetite	☐Normal, ☐↑, ☐↓
Weight	☐Normal, ☐↑, ☐↓; Past Wt.:_____ kg; Date:_____; Δ:_____
Thirst	☐Normal, ☐↑, ☐↓
Urination	☐Normal, ☐↑, ☐↓, ☐Blood, ☐Strain
Defecation	☐Normal, ☐↑, ☐↓, ☐Blood, ☐Strain, ☐Diarrhea, ☐Mucus
Discharge	☐No, ☐Yes; Onset/ Describe:
Cough/ Sneeze	☐No, ☐Yes; Onset/ Describe:
Vomit	☐No, ☐Yes; Onset/ Describe:
Respiration	☐Normal, ☐↑ Rate, ☐↑ Effort
Energy level	☐Normal, ☐Lethargic, ☐Exercise intolerance

• **Travel Hx**: ☐None, Other:_____
• **Exposure to**: ☐Standing water, ☐Wildlife, ☐Board/daycare, ☐Dog park, ☐Groomer, ☐Pet store
• **Adverse reactions to food/ meds**: ☐None, Other:_____
• **Can give oral meds**: ☐no ☐yes; Helpful Tricks:_____

Physical Exam – General:

- **Body Weight**:_____kg   **Body Condition Score**:____/9

- **Temperature**:_____°F [*Dog-RI*: 100.9–102.4; *Cat-RI*: 98.1–102.1]

- **Heart**:
  - *Rate*:_____beats/min [Dog-RI: 60–180; Cat-RI: 140–240 (in hospital)]
  - *Rhythm*: □Regular, □Irregular
  - *Sounds*: □None, □Split sound[S1 or S2], □Gallop[S3 or S4], □Murmur, □Muffled
    - *Grade*: □1–2[soft, only at PMI], □3–4[moderate, mild radiate], □5–6[loud, strong radiate, thrill]
    - *Timing*: □Systolic, □Diastolic, □Continuous
    - *PMI*:

	PMI	Over	Anatomic Boundaries
□	Lt. apex	Mitral valve	5th to 6th ICS at level of CCJ
□	Lt. base	Ao + Pul outflow	2nd to 4th ICS above the CCJ
□	Rt. midheart	Tricuspid valve	3rd to 5th ICS near the CCJ
□	Rt. sternal border	Right ventricle	5th to 7th ICS immediately dorsal to the sternum
□	Sternal (cat)	Sternum	In cats, determination of PMI offers very little clinical significance.

  - • *Vertebral Heart Size*: Dog = 8.7–10.7; Cat = 6.9–8.1 (from cranial edge of T4)
  - • *Innocent Murmur*: Grade 1-2, systolic, left base location, disappear by ~4 months of age, absent clinical signs

- **Pulses**:
  - *Pulse rate*:_____pulses/min
  - *Character*: □Sync, □Async; □Normokinetic, □Hyper-, □Hypo-, □Variable

- **Lungs**:
  - *Respiratory rate*:_____breaths/min [*RI*: 16–30]
  - *Depth/Effort*: □Norm, □Pant, □Deep, □Shallow, □↑ Insp. effort, □↑ Exp. effort
  - *Sounds/Localization*:
    - □Norm BV, □Quiet BV, □Loud BV, □Crack, □Wheez, □Frict, □Muffled
    - □All lung fields, □Rt cran, □Rt mid, □Rt caud, □Lt cran, □Lt mid, □Lt caud
  - *Tracheal Auscultation/ Palpation*: □Normal, Other:_____

- **Pain Score**:_____ / 5   Localization:_____

- **Mentation**: □BAR   □Confused/   □Drowsy/   □Stuporous   □Coma
  - □QAR   Disoriented   Obtunded   (unresponsive unless   (complete
  - □Dull   (conscious; inappropriate   (↓ interaction with   aroused by noxious   unresponsiveness
  - (conscious; responds   response to environment   environment; slow   stimuli)   to any stimuli)
  - to sensory stimuli)   [ex., vocalization, head   response to verbal
  - pressing])   stimuli)

- **Skin Elasticity**: □Normal skin turgor, □↓ Skin turgor, □Skin tent, □Gelatinous

- **Mucus Membranes**:
  - *CRT*:_____ [*RI*: 1–2; <1 = compensated shock, sepsis, heat stroke; <2 = acute decompensated shock; >2 = late decompensated shock, decreased cardiac output, hypothermia]
  - *Color*:_____ [*RI*: pink; red = compensated shock, sepsis, heat stroke; pale/white = anemia, shock; blue = cyanosis; yellow = hepatic disease, extravascular hemolysis; brown = met-Hb]
  - *Texture*:_____ [*RI*: moist = hydrated; tacky-to-dry = 5–12% dehydrated]

Physical Exam – Systems Checklist:

- Head:_____ □NAF
  - Ears: □Ceruminous debris (mild / mod / sev) (AS / AD / AU), _____ □NAF
  - Eyes:_____ □NAF
    - Retinal:_____ □NAF

→ Ⓛ	Ⓡ	Ⓛ	Ⓡ ←
□ ⊙ Normal Direct	□ ⊙ Normal Indirect	□ ⊙ Normal Indirect	□ ⊙ Normal Direct
□ ⊙ Abnormal Direct	□ ⊙ Abnormal Indirect	□ ⊙ Abnormal Indirect	□ ⊙ Abnormal Direct

  - Nose:_____ □NAF
  - Oral cavity: □Tarter/Gingivitis (mild / mod / sev), _____ □NAF
  - Mandibular lnn.: □Enlarged Lt., □Enlarged Rt., _____ □NAF

- Neck:_____ □NAF
  - Superficial cervical lnn.: □Enlarged Lt., □Enlarged Rt., _____ □NAF
  - Thyroid:_____ □NAF

- Thoracic limb:_____ □NAF
  - Foot pads:_____ □NAF
  - Knuckling:_____ □NAF
  - Axillary lnn. [normally absent]:_____ □NAF

- Thorax:_____ □NAF

- Abdomen:_____ □NAF
  - Mammary chain:_____ □NAF
  - Penis/ Testicles/ Vulva:_____ □NAF
  - Superficial inguinal lnn. [normally absent]:_____ □NAF

- Pelvic limb:_____ □NAF
  - Foot pads:_____ □NAF
  - Knuckling:_____ □NAF
  - Popliteal lnn.: □Enlarged Lt., □Enlarged Rt., _____ □NAF

- Skin:_____ □NAF
- Tail:_____ □NAF
- Rectal☞⊙:_____ □NAF

Problems List:

- **Problem #1**:

- **Problem #2**:

- **Problem #3**:

- **Problem #4**:

- **Problem #5**:

- **Problem #6**:

Diagnostic Plan	Treatment Plan

Case No._____

Patient	Age	Sex		Breed	Weight
		nM	sF		
	DOB:	iM	iF	Color:	kg

Owner	Primary Veterinarian	Admit Date/ Time
Name: Phone:	Name: Phone:	Date: Time: AM / PM

• **Presenting complaint**:_____

_____

_____

_____

_____

• **Medical Hx**:_____

_____

_____

_____

_____

• **When/ where obtained**: Date:_____; □Breeder, □Shelter, Other:_____

Drug/ Supplement	Amount	Dose (mg/kg)	Route	Frequency	Date Started

• **Vaccine status – Dog**: □Rab □Parv □Dist □Aden; □Para □Lep □Bord □Influ □Lyme
• **Vaccine status – Cat**: □Rab □Herp □Cali □Pan □FeLV [kittens]; □FIV □Chlam □Bord
• **Heartworm / Flea & Tick / Intestinal Parasites**:
  ○ *Last Heartworm Test*: Date:_____, □IDK; Test Results: □Pos, □Neg, □IDK
  ○ *Monthly heartworm preventative*: □no □yes, Product:_____
  ○ *Monthly flea & tick preventative*: □no □yes, Product:_____
  ○ *Monthly dewormer*:   □no □yes, Product:_____
• **Surgical Hx**: □Spay/Neuter; Date:_____; Other:_____
• **Environment**: □Indoor, □Outdoor, Time spent outdoors/ Other:_____
• **Housemates**: Dogs:_____ Cats:_____ Other:_____
• **Diet**: □Wet, □Dry; Brand/ Amt.:_____

Appetite	□Normal, □↑, □↓
Weight	□Normal, □↑, □↓; Past Wt.:_____ kg; Date:_____; Δ:_____
Thirst	□Normal, □↑, □↓
Urination	□Normal, □↑, □↓, □Blood, □Strain
Defecation	□Normal, □↑, □↓, □Blood, □Strain, □Diarrhea, □Mucus
Discharge	□No, □Yes; Onset/ Describe:
Cough/ Sneeze	□No, □Yes; Onset/ Describe:
Vomit	□No, □Yes; Onset/ Describe:
Respiration	□Normal, □↑ Rate, □↑ Effort
Energy level	□Normal, □Lethargic, □Exercise intolerance

• **Travel Hx**: □None, Other:_____
• **Exposure to**: □Standing water, □Wildlife, □Board/daycare, □Dog park, □Groomer, □Pet store
• **Adverse reactions to food/ meds**: □None, Other:_____
• **Can give oral meds**: □no □yes; Helpful Tricks:_____

Physical Exam – General:

- **Body Weight**:_____kg   **Body Condition Score**:___/9

- **Temperature**:_____°F [*Dog-RI*: 100.9–102.4; *Cat-RI*: 98.1–102.1]

- **Heart**:
  - *Rate*:_____beats/min [Dog-RI: 60–180; Cat-RI: 140–240 (in hospital)]
  - *Rhythm*: □Regular, □Irregular
  - *Sounds*: □None, □Split sound[S1 or S2], □Gallop[S3 or S4], □Murmur, □Muffled
    - *Grade*: □1–2[soft, only at PMI],   □3–4[moderate, mild radiate],   □5–6[loud, strong radiate, thrill]
    - *Timing*: □Systolic, □Diastolic, □Continuous
    - *PMI*:

	PMI	Over	Anatomic Boundaries
□	Lt. apex	Mitral valve	5th to 6th ICS at level of CCJ
□	Lt. base	Ao + Pul outflow	2nd to 4th ICS above the CCJ
□	Rt. midheart	Tricuspid valve	3rd to 5th ICS near the CCJ
□	Rt. sternal border	Right ventricle	5th to 7th ICS immediately dorsal to the sternum
□	Sternal (cat)	Sternum	In cats, determination of PMI offers very little clinical significance.

  - *Vertebral Heart Size*: Dog = 8.7–10.7; Cat = 6.9–8.1 (from cranial edge of T4)
  - *Innocent Murmur*: Grade 1-2, systolic, left base location, disappear by ~4 months of age, absent clinical signs

- **Pulses**:
  - *Pulse rate*:_____pulses/min
  - *Character*: □Sync, □Async;   □Normokinetic, □Hyper-, □Hypo-, □Variable

- **Lungs**:
  - *Respiratory rate*:_____breaths/min [*RI*: 16–30]
  - *Depth/Effort*: □Norm, □Pant, □Deep, □Shallow, □↑ Insp. effort, □↑ Exp. effort
  - *Sounds/Localization*:
    - □Norm BV, □Quiet BV, □Loud BV, □Crack, □Wheez, □Frict, □Muffled
    - □All lung fields, □Rt cran, □Rt mid, □Rt caud, □Lt cran, □Lt mid, □Lt caud
  - *Tracheal Auscultation/ Palpation*: □Normal, Other:_____

- **Pain Score**:_____ / 5   Localization:_____

- **Mentation**: □BAR   □Confused/   □Drowsy/   □Stuporous   □Coma
                 □QAR   Disoriented   Obtunded   (unresponsive unless   (complete
                 □Dull   (conscious; inappropriate   (↓ interaction with   aroused by noxious   unresponsiveness
                 (conscious; responds   response to environment   environment; slow   stimuli)   to any stimuli)
                 to sensory stimuli)   [ex., vocalization, head   response to verbal
                                       pressing])   stimuli)

- **Skin Elasticity**: □Normal skin turgor, □↓ Skin turgor, □Skin tent, □Gelatinous

- **Mucus Membranes**:
  - *CRT*:_____ [*RI*: 1–2; <1 = compensated shock, sepsis, heat stroke; <2 = acute decompensated shock; >2 = late decompensated shock, decreased cardiac output, hypothermia]
  - *Color*:_____ [*RI*: pink; red = compensated shock, sepsis, heat stroke; pale/white = anemia, shock; blue = cyanosis; yellow = hepatic disease, extravascular hemolysis; brown = met-Hb]
  - *Texture*:_____ [*RI*: moist = hydrated; tacky-to-dry = 5–12% dehydrated]

Physical Exam – Systems Checklist:

- Head: _____ ☐NAF
  - ○ Ears: ☐Ceruminous debris (mild / mod / sev) (AS / AD / AU), _____ ☐NAF
  - ○ Eyes: _____ ☐NAF
    - ▪ Retinal: _____ ☐NAF

→ Ⓛ		Ⓡ		Ⓛ		Ⓡ ←	
☐ ⊙ Normal Direct		☐ ⊙ Normal Indirect		☐ ⊙ Normal Indirect		☐ ⊙ Normal Direct	
☐ ● Abnormal Direct		☐ ● Abnormal Indirect		☐ ● Abnormal Indirect		☐ ● Abnormal Direct	

  - ○ Nose: _____ ☐NAF
  - ○ Oral cavity: ☐Tarter/Gingivitis (mild / mod / sev), _____ ☐NAF
  - ○ Mandibular lnn.: ☐Enlarged Lt., ☐Enlarged Rt., _____ ☐NAF

- Neck: _____ ☐NAF
  - ○ Superficial cervical lnn.: ☐Enlarged Lt., ☐Enlarged Rt., _____ ☐NAF
  - ○ Thyroid: _____ ☐NAF

- Thoracic limb: _____ ☐NAF
  - ○ Foot pads: _____ ☐NAF
  - ○ Knuckling: _____ ☐NAF
  - ○ Axillary lnn. [normally absent]: _____ ☐NAF

- Thorax: _____ ☐NAF

- Abdomen: _____ ☐NAF
  - ○ Mammary chain: _____ ☐NAF
  - ○ Penis/ Testicles/ Vulva: _____ ☐NAF
  - ○ Superficial inguinal lnn. [normally absent]: _____ ☐NAF

- Pelvic limb: _____ ☐NAF
  - ○ Foot pads: _____ ☐NAF
  - ○ Knuckling: _____ ☐NAF
  - ○ Popliteal lnn.: ☐Enlarged Lt., ☐Enlarged Rt., _____ ☐NAF

- Skin: _____ ☐NAF
- Tail: _____ ☐NAF
- Rectal☞⊙: _____ ☐NAF

Problems List:

• **Problem #1**:

• **Problem #2**:

• **Problem #3**:

• **Problem #4**:

• **Problem #5**:

• **Problem #6**:

Diagnostic Plan	Treatment Plan

Case No._____

Patient	Age	Sex		Breed	Weight
		nM	sF		
	DOB:	iM	iF	Color:	kg

Owner	Primary Veterinarian	Admit Date/ Time
Name: Phone:	Name: Phone:	Date: Time: AM / PM

• **Presenting complaint**:_____
_____
_____
_____
_____

• **Medical Hx**:_____
_____
_____
_____
_____

• **When/ where obtained**: Date:_____; ☐Breeder, ☐Shelter, Other:_____

Drug/ Supplement	Amount	Dose (mg/kg)	Route	Frequency	Date Started

• **Vaccine status – Dog**: ☐Rab ☐Parv ☐Dist ☐Aden; ☐Para ☐Lep ☐Bord ☐Influ ☐Lyme
• **Vaccine status – Cat**: ☐Rab ☐Herp ☐Cali ☐Pan ☐FeLV [kittens]; ☐FIV ☐Chlam ☐Bord
• **Heartworm / Flea & Tick / Intestinal Parasites**:
   ◦ *Last Heartworm Test*: Date:_____, ☐IDK; Test Results: ☐Pos, ☐Neg, ☐IDK
   ◦ *Monthly heartworm preventative*: ☐no ☐yes, Product:_____
   ◦ *Monthly flea & tick preventative*: ☐no ☐yes, Product:_____
   ◦ *Monthly dewormer*: ☐no ☐yes, Product:_____
• **Surgical Hx**: ☐Spay/Neuter; Date:_____; Other:_____
• **Environment**: ☐Indoor, ☐Outdoor, Time spent outdoors/ Other:_____
• **Housemates**: Dogs:_____ Cats:_____ Other:_____
• **Diet**: ☐Wet, ☐Dry; Brand/ Amt.:_____

Appetite	☐Normal, ☐↑, ☐↓
Weight	☐Normal, ☐↑, ☐↓; Past Wt.:_____ kg; Date:_____; Δ:_____
Thirst	☐Normal, ☐↑, ☐↓
Urination	☐Normal, ☐↑, ☐↓, ☐Blood, ☐Strain
Defecation	☐Normal, ☐↑, ☐↓, ☐Blood, ☐Strain, ☐Diarrhea, ☐Mucus
Discharge	☐No, ☐Yes; Onset/ Describe:
Cough/ Sneeze	☐No, ☐Yes; Onset/ Describe:
Vomit	☐No, ☐Yes; Onset/ Describe:
Respiration	☐Normal, ☐↑ Rate, ☐↑ Effort
Energy level	☐Normal, ☐Lethargic, ☐Exercise intolerance

• **Travel Hx**: ☐None, Other:_____
• **Exposure to**: ☐Standing water, ☐Wildlife, ☐Board/daycare, ☐Dog park, ☐Groomer, ☐Pet store
• **Adverse reactions to food/ meds**: ☐None, Other:_____
• **Can give oral meds**: ☐no ☐yes; Helpful Tricks:_____

Physical Exam – General:

- **Body Weight**:_____kg   **Body Condition Score**:____/9

- **Temperature**:_____°F [*Dog-RI*: 100.9–102.4; *Cat-RI*: 98.1–102.1]

- **Heart**:
  - *Rate*:_____beats/min [Dog-RI: 60–180; Cat-RI: 140–240 (in hospital)]
  - *Rhythm*: □Regular, □Irregular
  - *Sounds*: □None, □Split sound[S1 or S2], □Gallop[S3 or S4], □Murmur, □Muffled
    - *Grade*: □1–2[soft, only at PMI],   □3–4[moderate, mild radiate],   □5–6[loud, strong radiate, thrill]
    - *Timing*: □Systolic, □Diastolic, □Continuous
    - *PMI*:

	PMI	Over	Anatomic Boundaries
□	Lt. apex	Mitral valve	5th to 6th ICS at level of CCJ
□	Lt. base	Ao + Pul outflow	2nd to 4th ICS above the CCJ
□	Rt. midheart	Tricuspid valve	3rd to 5th ICS near the CCJ
□	Rt. sternal border	Right ventricle	5th to 7th ICS immediately dorsal to the sternum
□	Sternal (cat)	Sternum	In cats, determination of PMI offers very little clinical significance.

  - *Vertebral Heart Size*: Dog = 8.7–10.7; Cat = 6.9–8.1 (from cranial edge of T4)
  - *Innocent Murmur*: Grade 1-2, systolic, left base location, disappear by ~4 months of age, absent clinical signs

- **Pulses**:
  - *Pulse rate*:_____pulses/min
  - *Character*:   □Sync, □Async;   □Normokinetic, □Hyper-, □Hypo-, □Variable

- **Lungs**:
  - *Respiratory rate*:_____breaths/min [*RI*: 16–30]
  - *Depth/Effort*: □Norm, □Pant, □Deep, □Shallow, □↑ Insp. effort, □↑ Exp. effort
  - *Sounds/Localization*:
    - □Norm BV, □Quiet BV, □Loud BV, □Crack, □Wheez, □Frict, □Muffled
    - □All lung fields, □Rt cran, □Rt mid, □Rt caud, □Lt cran, □Lt mid, □Lt caud
  - *Tracheal Auscultation/ Palpation*: □Normal, Other:_____

- **Pain Score**:_____/ 5   Localization:_____

- **Mentation**:

□BAR	□Confused/	□Drowsy/	□Stuporous	□Coma
□QAR	Disoriented	Obtunded	(unresponsive unless aroused by noxious stimuli)	(complete unresponsiveness to any stimuli)
□Dull	(conscious; inappropriate response to environment [ex., vocalization, head pressing])	(↓ interaction with environment; slow response to verbal stimuli)		
(conscious; responds to sensory stimuli)				

- **Skin Elasticity**: □Normal skin turgor, □↓ Skin turgor, □Skin tent, □Gelatinous

- **Mucus Membranes**:
  - *CRT*:_____ [*RI*: 1–2; <1 = compensated shock, sepsis, heat stroke; <2 = acute decompensated shock; >2 = late decompensated shock, decreased cardiac output, hypothermia]
  - *Color*:_____ [*RI*: pink; red = compensated shock, sepsis, heat stroke; pale/white = anemia, shock; blue = cyanosis; yellow = hepatic disease, extravascular hemolysis; brown = met-Hb]
  - *Texture*:_____ [*RI*: moist = hydrated; tacky-to-dry = 5–12% dehydrated]

Physical Exam – Systems Checklist:

- Head:_____ ☐NAF
  - ○ Ears: ☐Ceruminous debris (mild / mod / sev) (AS / AD / AU), _____ ☐NAF
  - ○ Eyes:_____ ☐NAF
    - ▪ Retinal:_____ ☐NAF

→ Ⓛ		Ⓡ		Ⓛ		Ⓡ ←	
☐	⊙ Normal Direct	☐	⊙ Normal Indirect	☐	⊙ Normal Indirect	☐	⊙ Normal Direct
☐	● Abnormal Direct	☐	● Abnormal Indirect	☐	● Abnormal Indirect	☐	● Abnormal Direct

  - ○ Nose:_____ ☐NAF
  - ○ Oral cavity: ☐Tarter/Gingivitis (mild / mod / sev), _____ ☐NAF
  - ○ Mandibular lnn.: ☐Enlarged Lt., ☐Enlarged Rt., _____ ☐NAF

- Neck:_____ ☐NAF
  - ○ Superficial cervical lnn.: ☐Enlarged Lt., ☐Enlarged Rt., _____ ☐NAF
  - ○ Thyroid:_____ ☐NAF

- Thoracic limb:_____ ☐NAF
  - ○ Foot pads:_____ ☐NAF
  - ○ Knuckling:_____ ☐NAF
  - ○ Axillary lnn. [normally absent]:_____ ☐NAF

- Thorax:_____ ☐NAF

- Abdomen:_____ ☐NAF
  - ○ Mammary chain:_____ ☐NAF
  - ○ Penis/ Testicles/ Vulva:_____ ☐NAF
  - ○ Superficial inguinal lnn. [normally absent]:_____ ☐NAF

- Pelvic limb:_____ ☐NAF
  - ○ Foot pads:_____ ☐NAF
  - ○ Knuckling:_____ ☐NAF
  - ○ Popliteal lnn.: ☐Enlarged Lt., ☐Enlarged Rt., _____ ☐NAF

- Skin:_____ ☐NAF
- Tail:_____ ☐NAF
- Rectal☞☉:_____ ☐NAF

Problems List:

• **Problem #1**:

• **Problem #2**:

• **Problem #3**:

• **Problem #4**:

• **Problem #5**:

• **Problem #6**:

Diagnostic Plan	Treatment Plan

Case No._____

Patient	Age	Sex		Breed		Weight
		nM	sF			
	DOB:	iM	iF	Color:		kg

Owner	Primary Veterinarian	Admit Date/ Time
Name: Phone:	Name: Phone:	Date: Time: AM / PM

• **Presenting complaint**:_____
_____
_____
_____
_____
_____

• **Medical Hx**:_____
_____
_____
_____
_____

• **When/ where obtained**: Date:_____; ☐Breeder, ☐Shelter, Other:_____

Drug/ Supplement	Amount	Dose (mg/kg)	Route	Frequency	Date Started

• **Vaccine status – Dog**: ☐Rab ☐Parv ☐Dist ☐Aden; ☐Para ☐Lep ☐Bord ☐Influ ☐Lyme
• **Vaccine status – Cat**: ☐Rab ☐Herp ☐Cali ☐Pan ☐FeLV [kittens]; ☐FIV ☐Chlam ☐Bord
• **Heartworm / Flea & Tick / Intestinal Parasites**:
　○ *Last Heartworm Test*: Date:_____, ☐IDK; Test Results: ☐Pos, ☐Neg, ☐IDK
　○ *Monthly heartworm preventative*: ☐no ☐yes, Product:_____
　○ *Monthly flea & tick preventative*: ☐no ☐yes, Product:_____
　○ *Monthly dewormer*:　　　　　 ☐no ☐yes, Product:_____
• **Surgical Hx**: ☐Spay/Neuter; Date:_____; Other:_____
• **Environment**: ☐Indoor, ☐Outdoor, Time spent outdoors/ Other:_____
• **Housemates**: Dogs:_____ Cats:_____ Other:_____
• **Diet**: ☐Wet, ☐Dry; Brand/ Amt.:_____

Appetite	☐Normal, ☐↑, ☐↓
Weight	☐Normal, ☐↑, ☐↓; Past Wt.:_____ kg; Date:_____; Δ:_____
Thirst	☐Normal, ☐↑, ☐↓
Urination	☐Normal, ☐↑, ☐↓, ☐Blood, ☐Strain
Defecation	☐Normal, ☐↑, ☐↓, ☐Blood, ☐Strain, ☐Diarrhea, ☐Mucus
Discharge	☐No, ☐Yes; Onset/ Describe:
Cough/ Sneeze	☐No, ☐Yes; Onset/ Describe:
Vomit	☐No, ☐Yes; Onset/ Describe:
Respiration	☐Normal, ☐↑ Rate, ☐↑ Effort
Energy level	☐Normal, ☐Lethargic, ☐Exercise intolerance

• **Travel Hx**: ☐None, Other:_____
• **Exposure to**: ☐Standing water, ☐Wildlife, ☐Board/daycare, ☐Dog park, ☐Groomer, ☐Pet store
• **Adverse reactions to food/ meds**: ☐None, Other:_____
• **Can give oral meds**: ☐no ☐yes; Helpful Tricks:_____

Physical Exam – General:

- **Body Weight**:_____kg   **Body Condition Score**:____/9

- **Temperature**:_____°F [*Dog-RI*: 100.9–102.4;   *Cat-RI*: 98.1–102.1]

- **Heart**:
  - *Rate*:_____beats/min [Dog-RI: 60–180;   Cat-RI: 140–240 (in hospital)]
  - *Rhythm*: ☐Regular, ☐Irregular
  - *Sounds*: ☐None, ☐Split sound[S1 or S2], ☐Gallop[S3 or S4], ☐Murmur, ☐Muffled
    - *Grade*: ☐1–2[soft, only at PMI],   ☐3–4[moderate, mild radiate],   ☐5–6[loud, strong radiate, thrill]
    - *Timing*: ☐Systolic, ☐Diastolic, ☐Continuous
    - *PMI*:

	PMI	Over	Anatomic Boundaries
☐	Lt. apex	Mitral valve	5th to 6th ICS at level of CCJ
☐	Lt. base	Ao + Pul outflow	2nd to 4th ICS above the CCJ
☐	Rt. midheart	Tricuspid valve	3rd to 5th ICS near the CCJ
☐	Rt. sternal border	Right ventricle	5th to 7th ICS immediately dorsal to the sternum
☐	Sternal (cat)	Sternum	In cats, determination of PMI offers very little clinical significance.

  - •   *Vertebral Heart Size*: Dog = 8.7–10.7; Cat = 6.9–8.1 (from cranial edge of T4)
  - •   *Innocent Murmur*: Grade 1-2, systolic, left base location, disappear by ~4 months of age, absent clinical signs

- **Pulses**:
  - *Pulse rate*:_____pulses/min
  - *Character*: ☐Sync, ☐Async;   ☐Normokinetic, ☐Hyper-, ☐Hypo-, ☐Variable

- **Lungs**:
  - *Respiratory rate*:_____breaths/min [*RI*: 16–30]
  - *Depth/Effort*: ☐Norm, ☐Pant, ☐Deep, ☐Shallow, ☐↑ Insp. effort, ☐↑ Exp. effort
  - *Sounds/Localization*:
    - ☐Norm BV, ☐Quiet BV, ☐Loud BV, ☐Crack, ☐Wheez, ☐Frict, ☐Muffled
    - ☐All lung fields, ☐Rt cran, ☐Rt mid, ☐Rt caud, ☐Lt cran, ☐Lt mid, ☐Lt caud
  - *Tracheal Auscultation/ Palpation*: ☐Normal, Other:_____

- **Pain Score**:_____ / 5   Localization:_____

- **Mentation**:

☐BAR	☐Confused/	☐Drowsy/	☐Stuporous	☐Coma
☐QAR	Disoriented	Obtunded	(unresponsive unless aroused by noxious stimuli)	(complete unresponsiveness to any stimuli)
☐Dull	(conscious; inappropriate response to environment [ex., vocalization, head pressing])	(↓ interaction with environment; slow response to verbal stimuli)		
(conscious; responds to sensory stimuli)				

- **Skin Elasticity**: ☐Normal skin turgor, ☐↓ Skin turgor, ☐Skin tent, ☐Gelatinous

- **Mucus Membranes**:
  - *CRT*:_____ [*RI*: 1–2; <1 = compensated shock, sepsis, heat stroke; <2 = acute decompensated shock; >2 = late decompensated shock, decreased cardiac output, hypothermia]
  - *Color*:_____ [*RI*: pink; red = compensated shock, sepsis, heat stroke; pale/white = anemia, shock; blue = cyanosis; yellow = hepatic disease, extravascular hemolysis; brown = met-Hb]
  - *Texture*:_____ [*RI*: moist = hydrated; tacky-to-dry = 5–12% dehydrated]

Physical Exam – Systems Checklist:

- Head: _____ ☐NAF
  - Ears: ☐Ceruminous debris (mild / mod / sev) (AS / AD / AU), _____ ☐NAF
  - Eyes: _____ ☐NAF
    - Retinal: _____ ☐NAF

→ Ⓛ		Ⓡ		Ⓛ		Ⓡ ←	
☐	⊙ Normal Direct	☐	⊙ Normal Indirect	☐	⊙ Normal Indirect	☐	⊙ Normal Direct
☐	● Abnormal Direct	☐	● Abnormal Indirect	☐	● Abnormal Indirect	☐	● Abnormal Direct

  - Nose: _____ ☐NAF
  - Oral cavity: ☐Tarter/Gingivitis (mild / mod / sev), _____ ☐NAF
  - Mandibular lnn.: ☐Enlarged Lt., ☐Enlarged Rt., _____ ☐NAF

- Neck: _____ ☐NAF
  - Superficial cervical lnn.: ☐Enlarged Lt., ☐Enlarged Rt., _____ ☐NAF
  - Thyroid: _____ ☐NAF

- Thoracic limb: _____ ☐NAF
  - Foot pads: _____ ☐NAF
  - Knuckling: _____ ☐NAF
  - Axillary lnn. [normally absent]: _____ ☐NAF

- Thorax: _____ ☐NAF

- Abdomen: _____ ☐NAF
  - Mammary chain: _____ ☐NAF
  - Penis/ Testicles/ Vulva: _____ ☐NAF
  - Superficial inguinal lnn. [normally absent]: _____ ☐NAF

- Pelvic limb: _____ ☐NAF
  - Foot pads: _____ ☐NAF
  - Knuckling: _____ ☐NAF
  - Popliteal lnn.: ☐Enlarged Lt., ☐Enlarged Rt., _____ ☐NAF

- Skin: _____ ☐NAF
- Tail: _____ ☐NAF
- Rectal☞⊙: _____ ☐NAF

Problems List:

• **Problem #1**:

• **Problem #2**:

• **Problem #3**:

• **Problem #4**:

• **Problem #5**:

• **Problem #6**:

Diagnostic Plan	Treatment Plan

Case No._____

Patient	Age	Sex		Breed		Weight
		nM	sF			
	DOB:	iM	iF	Color:		kg

Owner	Primary Veterinarian	Admit Date/ Time
Name: Phone:	Name: Phone:	Date: Time: AM / PM

• **Presenting complaint**:_____
_____
_____
_____
_____
_____

• **Medical Hx**:_____
_____
_____
_____
_____

• **When/ where obtained**: Date:_____; ☐Breeder, ☐Shelter, Other:_____

Drug/ Supplement	Amount	Dose (mg/kg)	Route	Frequency	Date Started

• **Vaccine status – Dog**: ☐Rab ☐Parv ☐Dist ☐Aden; ☐Para ☐Lep ☐Bord ☐Influ ☐Lyme
• **Vaccine status – Cat**: ☐Rab ☐Herp ☐Cali ☐Pan ☐FeLV [kittens]; ☐FIV ☐Chlam ☐Bord
• **Heartworm / Flea & Tick / Intestinal Parasites**:
   ◦ *Last Heartworm Test*: Date:_____, ☐IDK; Test Results: ☐Pos, ☐Neg, ☐IDK
   ◦ *Monthly heartworm preventative*: ☐no ☐yes, Product:_____
   ◦ *Monthly flea & tick preventative*: ☐no ☐yes, Product:_____
   ◦ *Monthly dewormer*:   ☐no ☐yes, Product:_____
• **Surgical Hx**: ☐Spay/Neuter; Date:_____; Other:_____
• **Environment**: ☐Indoor, ☐Outdoor, Time spent outdoors/ Other:_____
• **Housemates**: Dogs:_____ Cats:_____ Other:_____
• **Diet**: ☐Wet, ☐Dry; Brand/ Amt.:_____

Appetite	☐Normal, ☐↑, ☐↓
Weight	☐Normal, ☐↑, ☐↓; Past Wt.:_____ kg; Date:_____; Δ:_____
Thirst	☐Normal, ☐↑, ☐↓
Urination	☐Normal, ☐↑, ☐↓, ☐Blood, ☐Strain
Defecation	☐Normal, ☐↑, ☐↓, ☐Blood, ☐Strain, ☐Diarrhea, ☐Mucus
Discharge	☐No, ☐Yes; Onset/ Describe:
Cough/ Sneeze	☐No, ☐Yes; Onset/ Describe:
Vomit	☐No, ☐Yes; Onset/ Describe:
Respiration	☐Normal, ☐↑ Rate, ☐↑ Effort
Energy level	☐Normal, ☐Lethargic, ☐Exercise intolerance

• **Travel Hx**: ☐None, Other:_____
• **Exposure to**: ☐Standing water, ☐Wildlife, ☐Board/daycare, ☐Dog park, ☐Groomer, ☐Pet store
• **Adverse reactions to food/ meds**: ☐None, Other:_____
• **Can give oral meds**: ☐no ☐yes; Helpful Tricks:_____

Physical Exam – General:

- **Body Weight:**_____ kg   **Body Condition Score:**____/9

- **Temperature:**_____ °F [*Dog-RI*: 100.9–102.4;   *Cat-RI*: 98.1–102.1]

- **Heart:**
  - *Rate:*_____ beats/min [Dog-RI: 60–180;   Cat-RI: 140–240 (in hospital)]
  - *Rhythm:* ☐Regular, ☐Irregular
  - *Sounds:* ☐None, ☐Split sound[S1 or S2], ☐Gallop[S3 or S4], ☐Murmur, ☐Muffled
    - *Grade:* ☐1–2[soft, only at PMI],   ☐3–4[moderate, mild radiate],   ☐5–6[loud, strong radiate, thrill]
    - *Timing:* ☐Systolic, ☐Diastolic, ☐Continuous
    - *PMI:*

	PMI	Over	Anatomic Boundaries
☐	Lt. apex	Mitral valve	5th to 6th ICS at level of CCJ
☐	Lt. base	Ao + Pul outflow	2nd to 4th ICS above the CCJ
☐	Rt. midheart	Tricuspid valve	3rd to 5th ICS near the CCJ
☐	Rt. sternal border	Right ventricle	5th to 7th ICS immediately dorsal to the sternum
☐	Sternal (cat)	Sternum	In cats, determination of PMI offers very little clinical significance.

  - • *Vertebral Heart Size*: Dog = 8.7–10.7; Cat = 6.9–8.1 (from cranial edge of T4)
  - • *Innocent Murmur*: Grade 1-2, systolic, left base location, disappear by ~4 months of age, absent clinical signs

- **Pulses:**
  - *Pulse rate:*_____ pulses/min
  - *Character:* ☐Sync, ☐Async;   ☐Normokinetic, ☐Hyper-, ☐Hypo-, ☐Variable

- **Lungs:**
  - *Respiratory rate:*_____ breaths/min [*RI*: 16–30]
  - *Depth/Effort:* ☐Norm, ☐Pant, ☐Deep, ☐Shallow, ☐↑ Insp. effort, ☐↑ Exp. effort
  - *Sounds/Localization:*
    - ☐Norm BV, ☐Quiet BV, ☐Loud BV, ☐Crack, ☐Wheez, ☐Frict, ☐Muffled
    - ☐All lung fields, ☐Rt cran, ☐Rt mid, ☐Rt caud, ☐Lt cran, ☐Lt mid, ☐Lt caud
  - *Tracheal Auscultation/ Palpation:* ☐Normal, Other:_____

- **Pain Score:**_____ / 5   Localization:_____

- **Mentation:** ☐BAR   ☐Confused/   ☐Drowsy/   ☐Stuporous   ☐Coma
  - ☐QAR   Disoriented   Obtunded   (unresponsive unless   (complete
  - ☐Dull   (conscious; inappropriate   (↓ interaction with   aroused by noxious   unresponsiveness
  - (conscious; responds   response to environment   environment; slow   stimuli)   to any stimuli)
  - to sensory stimuli)   [ex., vocalization, head   response to verbal
  -     pressing])   stimuli)

- **Skin Elasticity:** ☐Normal skin turgor, ☐↓ Skin turgor, ☐Skin tent, ☐Gelatinous

- **Mucus Membranes:**
  - *CRT:*_____ [*RI*: 1–2; <1 = compensated shock, sepsis, heat stroke; <2 = acute decompensated shock; >2 = late decompensated shock, decreased cardiac output, hypothermia]
  - *Color:*_____ [*RI*: pink; red = compensated shock, sepsis, heat stroke; pale/white = anemia, shock; blue = cyanosis; yellow = hepatic disease, extravascular hemolysis; brown = met-Hb]
  - *Texture:*_____ [*RI*: moist = hydrated; tacky-to-dry = 5–12% dehydrated]

Physical Exam – Systems Checklist:

- Head:_____ ☐NAF
  - Ears: ☐Ceruminous debris (mild / mod / sev) (AS / AD / AU), _____ ☐NAF
  - Eyes:_____ ☐NAF
    - Retinal:_____ ☐NAF

→ Ⓛ	Ⓡ	Ⓛ	Ⓡ ←
☐ ⊙ Normal Direct	☐ ⊙ Normal Indirect	☐ ⊙ Normal Indirect	☐ ⊙ Normal Direct
☐ ⦿ Abnormal Direct	☐ ⦿ Abnormal Indirect	☐ ⦿ Abnormal Indirect	☐ ⦿ Abnormal Direct

  - Nose:_____ ☐NAF
  - Oral cavity: ☐Tarter/Gingivitis (mild / mod / sev), _____ ☐NAF
  - Mandibular lnn.: ☐Enlarged Lt., ☐Enlarged Rt., _____ ☐NAF

- Neck:_____ ☐NAF
  - Superficial cervical lnn.: ☐Enlarged Lt., ☐Enlarged Rt., _____ ☐NAF
  - Thyroid:_____ ☐NAF

- Thoracic limb:_____ ☐NAF
  - Foot pads:_____ ☐NAF
  - Knuckling:_____ ☐NAF
  - Axillary lnn. [normally absent]:_____ ☐NAF

- Thorax:_____ ☐NAF

- Abdomen:_____ ☐NAF
  - Mammary chain:_____ ☐NAF
  - Penis/ Testicles/ Vulva:_____ ☐NAF
  - Superficial inguinal lnn. [normally absent]:_____ ☐NAF

- Pelvic limb:_____ ☐NAF
  - Foot pads:_____ ☐NAF
  - Knuckling:_____ ☐NAF
  - Popliteal lnn.: ☐Enlarged Lt., ☐Enlarged Rt., _____ ☐NAF

- Skin:_____ ☐NAF
- Tail:_____ ☐NAF
- Rectal☞☉:_____ ☐NAF

Problems List:

- **Problem #1**:

- **Problem #2**:

- **Problem #3**:

- **Problem #4**:

- **Problem #5**:

- **Problem #6**:

Diagnostic Plan	Treatment Plan

Case No._____

Patient	Age	Sex		Breed	Weight
		nM	sF		
	DOB:	iM	iF	Color:	kg

Owner	Primary Veterinarian	Admit Date/ Time
Name: Phone:	Name: Phone:	Date: Time: AM / PM

• **Presenting complaint**:_____
_____
_____
_____
_____
_____

• **Medical Hx**:_____
_____
_____
_____
_____

• **When/ where obtained**: Date:_____; ☐Breeder, ☐Shelter, Other:_____

Drug/ Supplement	Amount	Dose (mg/kg)	Route	Frequency	Date Started

• **Vaccine status – Dog**: ☐Rab ☐Parv ☐Dist ☐Aden; ☐Para ☐Lep ☐Bord ☐Influ ☐Lyme
• **Vaccine status – Cat**: ☐Rab ☐Herp ☐Cali ☐Pan ☐FeLV [kittens]; ☐FIV ☐Chlam ☐Bord
• **Heartworm / Flea & Tick / Intestinal Parasites**:
  ◦ *Last Heartworm Test*: Date:_____, ☐IDK; Test Results: ☐Pos, ☐Neg, ☐IDK
  ◦ *Monthly heartworm preventative*: ☐no ☐yes, Product:_____
  ◦ *Monthly flea & tick preventative*: ☐no ☐yes, Product:_____
  ◦ *Monthly dewormer*: ☐no ☐yes, Product:_____
• **Surgical Hx**: ☐Spay/Neuter; Date:_____; Other:_____
• **Environment**: ☐Indoor, ☐Outdoor, Time spent outdoors/ Other:_____
• **Housemates**: Dogs:_____ Cats:_____ Other:_____
• **Diet**: ☐Wet, ☐Dry; Brand/ Amt.:_____

Appetite	☐Normal, ☐↑, ☐↓
Weight	☐Normal, ☐↑, ☐↓; Past Wt.:_____ kg; Date:_____; Δ:_____
Thirst	☐Normal, ☐↑, ☐↓
Urination	☐Normal, ☐↑, ☐↓, ☐Blood, ☐Strain
Defecation	☐Normal, ☐↑, ☐↓, ☐Blood, ☐Strain, ☐Diarrhea, ☐Mucus
Discharge	☐No, ☐Yes; Onset/ Describe:
Cough/ Sneeze	☐No, ☐Yes; Onset/ Describe:
Vomit	☐No, ☐Yes; Onset/ Describe:
Respiration	☐Normal, ☐↑ Rate, ☐↑ Effort
Energy level	☐Normal, ☐Lethargic, ☐Exercise intolerance

• **Travel Hx**: ☐None, Other:_____
• **Exposure to**: ☐Standing water, ☐Wildlife, ☐Board/daycare, ☐Dog park, ☐Groomer, ☐Pet store
• **Adverse reactions to food/ meds**: ☐None, Other:_____
• **Can give oral meds**: ☐no ☐yes; Helpful Tricks:_____

Physical Exam – General:

- **Body Weight**:_____ kg   **Body Condition Score**:___/9

- **Temperature**:_____ °F [*Dog-RI*: 100.9–102.4; *Cat-RI*: 98.1–102.1]

- **Heart**:
  - *Rate*:_____ beats/min [Dog-RI: 60–180; Cat-RI: 140–240 (in hospital)]
  - *Rhythm*: □Regular, □Irregular
  - *Sounds*: □None, □Split sound[S1 or S2], □Gallop[S3 or S4], □Murmur, □Muffled
    - *Grade*: □1–2[soft, only at PMI],   □3–4[moderate, mild radiate],   □5–6[loud, strong radiate, thrill]
    - *Timing*: □Systolic, □Diastolic, □Continuous
    - *PMI*:

	PMI	Over	Anatomic Boundaries
□	Lt. apex	Mitral valve	5th to 6th ICS at level of CCJ
□	Lt. base	Ao + Pul outflow	2nd to 4th ICS above the CCJ
□	Rt. midheart	Tricuspid valve	3rd to 5th ICS near the CCJ
□	Rt. sternal border	Right ventricle	5th to 7th ICS immediately dorsal to the sternum
□	Sternal (cat)	Sternum	In cats, determination of PMI offers very little clinical significance.

- *Vertebral Heart Size*: Dog = 8.7–10.7; Cat = 6.9–8.1 (from cranial edge of T4)
- *Innocent Murmur*: Grade 1-2, systolic, left base location, disappear by ~4 months of age, absent clinical signs

- **Pulses**:
  - *Pulse rate*:_____ pulses/min
  - *Character*:   □Sync, □Async;   □Normokinetic, □Hyper-, □Hypo-, □Variable

- **Lungs**:
  - *Respiratory rate*:_____ breaths/min [*RI*: 16–30]
  - *Depth/Effort*: □Norm, □Pant, □Deep, □Shallow, □↑ Insp. effort, □↑ Exp. effort
  - *Sounds/Localization*:
    - □Norm BV, □Quiet BV, □Loud BV, □Crack, □Wheez, □Frict, □Muffled
    - □All lung fields, □Rt cran, □Rt mid, □Rt caud, □Lt cran, □Lt mid, □Lt caud
  - *Tracheal Auscultation/ Palpation*: □Normal, Other:_____

- **Pain Score**:_____ / 5   Localization:_____

- **Mentation**: □BAR   □Confused/   □Drowsy/   □Stuporous   □Coma
  □QAR   Disoriented   Obtunded   (unresponsive unless   (complete
  □Dull   (conscious; inappropriate   (↓ interaction with   aroused by noxious   unresponsiveness
  (conscious; responds   response to environment   environment; slow   stimuli)   to any stimuli)
  to sensory stimuli)   [ex., vocalization, head   response to verbal
  pressing])   stimuli)

- **Skin Elasticity**: □Normal skin turgor, □↓ Skin turgor, □Skin tent, □Gelatinous

- **Mucus Membranes**:
  - *CRT*:_____ [*RI*: 1–2; <1 = compensated shock, sepsis, heat stroke; <2 = acute decompensated shock; >2 = late decompensated shock, decreased cardiac output, hypothermia]
  - *Color*:_____ [*RI*: pink; red = compensated shock, sepsis, heat stroke; pale/white = anemia, shock; blue = cyanosis; yellow = hepatic disease, extravascular hemolysis; brown = met-Hb]
  - *Texture*:_____ [*RI*: moist = hydrated; tacky-to-dry = 5–12% dehydrated]

Physical Exam – Systems Checklist:

- Head:_____ ☐NAF
  - ◦ Ears: ☐Ceruminous debris (mild / mod / sev) (AS / AD / AU), _____ ☐NAF
  - ◦ Eyes:_____ ☐NAF
    - ▪ Retinal:_____ ☐NAF

→ Ⓛ		Ⓡ		Ⓛ		Ⓡ ←	
☐	⊙ Normal Direct	☐	⊙ Normal Indirect	☐	⊙ Normal Indirect	☐	⊙ Normal Direct
☐	⊙ Abnormal Direct	☐	⊙ Abnormal Indirect	☐	⊙ Abnormal Indirect	☐	⊙ Abnormal Direct

  - ◦ Nose:_____ ☐NAF
  - ◦ Oral cavity: ☐Tarter/Gingivitis (mild / mod / sev), _____ ☐NAF
  - ◦ Mandibular lnn.: ☐Enlarged Lt., ☐Enlarged Rt., _____ ☐NAF

- Neck:_____ ☐NAF
  - ◦ Superficial cervical lnn.: ☐Enlarged Lt., ☐Enlarged Rt., _____ ☐NAF
  - ◦ Thyroid:_____ ☐NAF

- Thoracic limb:_____ ☐NAF
  - ◦ Foot pads:_____ ☐NAF
  - ◦ Knuckling:_____ ☐NAF
  - ◦ Axillary lnn. [normally absent]:_____ ☐NAF

- Thorax:_____ ☐NAF

- Abdomen:_____ ☐NAF
  - ◦ Mammary chain:_____ ☐NAF
  - ◦ Penis/ Testicles/ Vulva:_____ ☐NAF
  - ◦ Superficial inguinal lnn. [normally absent]:_____ ☐NAF

- Pelvic limb:_____ ☐NAF
  - ◦ Foot pads:_____ ☐NAF
  - ◦ Knuckling:_____ ☐NAF
  - ◦ Popliteal lnn.: ☐Enlarged Lt., ☐Enlarged Rt., _____ ☐NAF

- Skin:_____ ☐NAF
- Tail:_____ ☐NAF
- Rectal☞☉:_____ ☐NAF

Problems List:

- **Problem #1**:

- **Problem #2**:

- **Problem #3**:

- **Problem #4**:

- **Problem #5**:

- **Problem #6**:

Diagnostic Plan	Treatment Plan

Case No._____

Patient	Age	Sex		Breed		Weight
		nM	sF			
	DOB:	iM	iF	Color:		kg

Owner	Primary Veterinarian	Admit Date/ Time
Name: Phone:	Name: Phone:	Date: Time: AM / PM

• Presenting complaint:_____
_____
_____
_____
_____
_____

• Medical Hx:_____
_____
_____
_____
_____

• When/ where obtained: Date:_____; ☐Breeder, ☐Shelter, Other:_____

Drug/ Supplement	Amount	Dose (mg/kg)	Route	Frequency	Date Started

• Vaccine status – Dog: ☐Rab ☐Parv ☐Dist ☐Aden; ☐Para ☐Lep ☐Bord ☐Influ ☐Lyme
• Vaccine status – Cat: ☐Rab ☐Herp ☐Cali ☐Pan ☐FeLV [kittens]; ☐FIV ☐Chlam ☐Bord
• Heartworm / Flea & Tick / Intestinal Parasites:
  ◦ *Last Heartworm Test*: Date:_____, ☐IDK; Test Results: ☐Pos, ☐Neg, ☐IDK
  ◦ *Monthly heartworm preventative*: ☐no ☐yes, Product:_____
  ◦ *Monthly flea & tick preventative*: ☐no ☐yes, Product:_____
  ◦ *Monthly dewormer*:   ☐no ☐yes, Product:_____
• Surgical Hx: ☐Spay/Neuter; Date:_____; Other:_____
• Environment: ☐Indoor, ☐Outdoor, Time spent outdoors/ Other:_____
• Housemates: Dogs:_____ Cats:_____ Other:_____
• Diet: ☐Wet, ☐Dry; Brand/ Amt.:_____

Appetite	☐Normal, ☐↑, ☐↓
Weight	☐Normal, ☐↑, ☐↓; Past Wt.:_____ kg; Date:_____; Δ:_____
Thirst	☐Normal, ☐↑, ☐↓
Urination	☐Normal, ☐↑, ☐↓, ☐Blood, ☐Strain
Defecation	☐Normal, ☐↑, ☐↓, ☐Blood, ☐Strain, ☐Diarrhea, ☐Mucus
Discharge	☐No, ☐Yes; Onset/ Describe:
Cough/ Sneeze	☐No, ☐Yes; Onset/ Describe:
Vomit	☐No, ☐Yes; Onset/ Describe:
Respiration	☐Normal, ☐↑ Rate, ☐↑ Effort
Energy level	☐Normal, ☐Lethargic, ☐Exercise intolerance

• Travel Hx: ☐None, Other:_____
• Exposure to: ☐Standing water, ☐Wildlife, ☐Board/daycare, ☐Dog park, ☐Groomer, ☐Pet store
• Adverse reactions to food/ meds: ☐None, Other:_____
• Can give oral meds: ☐no ☐yes; Helpful Tricks:_____

Physical Exam – General:

- **Body Weight**:_____kg   **Body Condition Score**:___/9

- **Temperature**:_____°F [*Dog-RI*: 100.9–102.4; *Cat-RI*: 98.1–102.1]

- **Heart**:
  - *Rate*:_____beats/min [Dog-RI: 60–180; Cat-RI: 140–240 (in hospital)]
  - *Rhythm*: ☐Regular, ☐Irregular
  - *Sounds*: ☐None, ☐Split sound[S1 or S2], ☐Gallop[S3 or S4], ☐Murmur, ☐Muffled
    - *Grade*: ☐1–2[soft, only at PMI], ☐3–4[moderate, mild radiate], ☐5–6[loud, strong radiate, thrill]
    - *Timing*: ☐Systolic, ☐Diastolic, ☐Continuous
    - *PMI*:

	PMI	Over	Anatomic Boundaries
☐	Lt. apex	Mitral valve	5th to 6th ICS at level of CCJ
☐	Lt. base	Ao + Pul outflow	2nd to 4th ICS above the CCJ
☐	Rt. midheart	Tricuspid valve	3rd to 5th ICS near the CCJ
☐	Rt. sternal border	Right ventricle	5th to 7th ICS immediately dorsal to the sternum
☐	Sternal (cat)	Sternum	In cats, determination of PMI offers very little clinical significance.

  - • *Vertebral Heart Size*: Dog = 8.7–10.7; Cat = 6.9–8.1 (from cranial edge of T4)
  - • *Innocent Murmur*: Grade 1-2, systolic, left base location, disappear by ~4 months of age, absent clinical signs

- **Pulses**:
  - *Pulse rate*:_____pulses/min
  - *Character*: ☐Sync, ☐Async; ☐Normokinetic, ☐Hyper-, ☐Hypo-, ☐Variable

- **Lungs**:
  - *Respiratory rate*:_____breaths/min [*RI*: 16–30]
  - *Depth/Effort*: ☐Norm, ☐Pant, ☐Deep, ☐Shallow, ☐↑ Insp. effort, ☐↑ Exp. effort
  - *Sounds/Localization*:
    - ☐Norm BV, ☐Quiet BV, ☐Loud BV, ☐Crack, ☐Wheez, ☐Frict, ☐Muffled
    - ☐All lung fields, ☐Rt cran, ☐Rt mid, ☐Rt caud, ☐Lt cran, ☐Lt mid, ☐Lt caud
  - *Tracheal Auscultation/ Palpation*: ☐Normal, Other:_____

- **Pain Score**:_____ / 5   Localization:_____

- **Mentation**: ☐BAR   ☐Confused/   ☐Drowsy/   ☐Stuporous   ☐Coma

  ☐QAR   Disoriented   Obtunded   (unresponsive unless   (complete

  ☐Dull   (conscious; inappropriate   (↓ interaction with   aroused by noxious   unresponsiveness

  (conscious; responds   response to environment   environment; slow   stimuli)   to any stimuli)

  to sensory stimuli)   [ex., vocalization, head   response to verbal

  pressing])   stimuli)

- **Skin Elasticity**: ☐Normal skin turgor, ☐↓ Skin turgor, ☐Skin tent, ☐Gelatinous

- **Mucus Membranes**:
  - *CRT*:_____ [*RI*: 1–2; <1 = compensated shock, sepsis, heat stroke; <2 = acute decompensated shock; >2 = late decompensated shock, decreased cardiac output, hypothermia]
  - *Color*:_____ [*RI*: pink; red = compensated shock, sepsis, heat stroke; pale/white = anemia, shock; blue = cyanosis; yellow = hepatic disease, extravascular hemolysis; brown = met-Hb]
  - *Texture*:_____ [*RI*: moist = hydrated; tacky-to-dry = 5–12% dehydrated]

Physical Exam – Systems Checklist:

- **Head:** _____ ☐NAF
  - Ears: ☐Ceruminous debris (mild / mod / sev) (AS / AD / AU), _____ ☐NAF
  - Eyes: _____ ☐NAF
    - Retinal: _____ ☐NAF

→ Ⓛ		Ⓡ		Ⓛ		Ⓡ ←	
☐	⊙ Normal Direct	☐	⊙ Normal Indirect	☐	⊙ Normal Indirect	☐	⊙ Normal Direct
☐	⊙ Abnormal Direct	☐	⊙ Abnormal Indirect	☐	⊙ Abnormal Indirect	☐	⊙ Abnormal Direct

  - Nose: _____ ☐NAF
  - Oral cavity: ☐Tarter/Gingivitis (mild / mod / sev), _____ ☐NAF
  - Mandibular lnn.: ☐Enlarged Lt., ☐Enlarged Rt., _____ ☐NAF

- **Neck:** _____ ☐NAF
  - Superficial cervical lnn.: ☐Enlarged Lt., ☐Enlarged Rt., _____ ☐NAF
  - Thyroid: _____ ☐NAF

- **Thoracic limb:** _____ ☐NAF
  - Foot pads: _____ ☐NAF
  - Knuckling: _____ ☐NAF
  - Axillary lnn. [normally absent]: _____ ☐NAF

- **Thorax:** _____ ☐NAF

- **Abdomen:** _____ ☐NAF
  - Mammary chain: _____ ☐NAF
  - Penis/ Testicles/ Vulva: _____ ☐NAF
  - Superficial inguinal lnn. [normally absent]: _____ ☐NAF

- **Pelvic limb:** _____ ☐NAF
  - Foot pads: _____ ☐NAF
  - Knuckling: _____ ☐NAF
  - Popliteal lnn.: ☐Enlarged Lt., ☐Enlarged Rt., _____ ☐NAF

- **Skin:** _____ ☐NAF
- **Tail:** _____ ☐NAF
- **Rectal☞⊙:** _____ ☐NAF

Problems List:

• **Problem #1**:

• **Problem #2**:

• **Problem #3**:

• **Problem #4**:

• **Problem #5**:

• **Problem #6**:

Diagnostic Plan	Treatment Plan

Case No._____

Patient	Age	Sex		Breed		Weight
		nM	sF			
	DOB:	iM	iF	Color:		kg

Owner	Primary Veterinarian	Admit Date/ Time
Name: Phone:	Name: Phone:	Date: Time: AM / PM

• **Presenting complaint**:_____
_____
_____
_____
_____
_____

• **Medical Hx**:_____
_____
_____
_____
_____

• **When/ where obtained**: Date:_____; ☐Breeder, ☐Shelter, Other:_____

Drug/ Supplement	Amount	Dose (mg/kg)	Route	Frequency	Date Started

• **Vaccine status – Dog**: ☐Rab ☐Parv ☐Dist ☐Aden; ☐Para ☐Lep ☐Bord ☐Influ ☐Lyme
• **Vaccine status – Cat**: ☐Rab ☐Herp ☐Cali ☐Pan ☐FeLV [kittens]; ☐FIV ☐Chlam ☐Bord
• **Heartworm / Flea & Tick / Intestinal Parasites**:
　◦ *Last Heartworm Test*: Date:_____, ☐IDK; Test Results: ☐Pos, ☐Neg, ☐IDK
　◦ *Monthly heartworm preventative*: ☐no ☐yes, Product:_____
　◦ *Monthly flea & tick preventative*: ☐no ☐yes, Product:_____
　◦ *Monthly dewormer*: ☐no ☐yes, Product:_____
• **Surgical Hx**: ☐Spay/Neuter; Date:_____; Other:_____
• **Environment**: ☐Indoor, ☐Outdoor, Time spent outdoors/ Other:_____
• **Housemates**: Dogs:_____ Cats:_____ Other:_____
• **Diet**: ☐Wet, ☐Dry; Brand/ Amt.:_____

Appetite	☐Normal, ☐↑, ☐↓
Weight	☐Normal, ☐↑, ☐↓; Past Wt.:_____ kg; Date:_____; Δ:_____
Thirst	☐Normal, ☐↑, ☐↓
Urination	☐Normal, ☐↑, ☐↓, ☐Blood, ☐Strain
Defecation	☐Normal, ☐↑, ☐↓, ☐Blood, ☐Strain, ☐Diarrhea, ☐Mucus
Discharge	☐No, ☐Yes; Onset/ Describe:
Cough/ Sneeze	☐No, ☐Yes; Onset/ Describe:
Vomit	☐No, ☐Yes; Onset/ Describe:
Respiration	☐Normal, ☐↑ Rate, ☐↑ Effort
Energy level	☐Normal, ☐Lethargic, ☐Exercise intolerance

• **Travel Hx**: ☐None, Other:_____
• **Exposure to**: ☐Standing water, ☐Wildlife, ☐Board/daycare, ☐Dog park, ☐Groomer, ☐Pet store
• **Adverse reactions to food/ meds**: ☐None, Other:_____
• **Can give oral meds**: ☐no ☐yes; Helpful Tricks:_____

Physical Exam – General:

- **Body Weight**:_____kg **Body Condition Score**:___/9

- **Temperature**:_____°F [*Dog-RI*: 100.9–102.4; *Cat-RI*: 98.1–102.1]

- **Heart**:
  - *Rate*:_____beats/min [Dog-RI: 60–180; Cat-RI: 140–240 (in hospital)]
  - *Rhythm*: ☐Regular, ☐Irregular
  - *Sounds*: ☐None, ☐Split sound[S1 or S2], ☐Gallop[S3 or S4], ☐Murmur, ☐Muffled
    - *Grade*: ☐1–2[soft, only at PMI], ☐3–4[moderate, mild radiate], ☐5–6[loud, strong radiate, thrill]
    - *Timing*: ☐Systolic, ☐Diastolic, ☐Continuous
    - *PMI*:

	PMI	Over	Anatomic Boundaries
☐	Lt. apex	Mitral valve	5th to 6th ICS at level of CCJ
☐	Lt. base	Ao + Pul outflow	2nd to 4th ICS above the CCJ
☐	Rt. midheart	Tricuspid valve	3rd to 5th ICS near the CCJ
☐	Rt. sternal border	Right ventricle	5th to 7th ICS immediately dorsal to the sternum
☐	Sternal (cat)	Sternum	In cats, determination of PMI offers very little clinical significance.

  - *Vertebral Heart Size*: Dog = 8.7–10.7; Cat = 6.9–8.1 (from cranial edge of T4)
  - *Innocent Murmur*: Grade 1-2, systolic, left base location, disappear by ~4 months of age, absent clinical signs

- **Pulses**:
  - *Pulse rate*:_____pulses/min
  - *Character*: ☐Sync, ☐Async; ☐Normokinetic, ☐Hyper-, ☐Hypo-, ☐Variable

- **Lungs**:
  - *Respiratory rate*:_____breaths/min [RI: 16–30]
  - *Depth/Effort*: ☐Norm, ☐Pant, ☐Deep, ☐Shallow, ☐↑ Insp. effort, ☐↑ Exp. effort
  - *Sounds/Localization*:
    - ☐Norm BV, ☐Quiet BV, ☐Loud BV, ☐Crack, ☐Wheez, ☐Frict, ☐Muffled
    - ☐All lung fields, ☐Rt cran, ☐Rt mid, ☐Rt caud, ☐Lt cran, ☐Lt mid, ☐Lt caud
  - *Tracheal Auscultation/ Palpation*: ☐Normal, Other:_____

- **Pain Score**:_____ / 5   Localization:_____

- **Mentation**: ☐BAR   ☐Confused/   ☐Drowsy/   ☐Stuporous   ☐Coma
  ☐QAR   Disoriented   Obtunded   (unresponsive unless   (complete
  ☐Dull   (conscious; inappropriate   (↓ interaction with   aroused by noxious   unresponsiveness
  (conscious; responds   response to environment   environment; slow   stimuli)   to any stimuli)
  to sensory stimuli)   [ex., vocalization, head   response to verbal
  pressing])   stimuli)

- **Skin Elasticity**: ☐Normal skin turgor, ☐↓ Skin turgor, ☐Skin tent, ☐Gelatinous

- **Mucus Membranes**:
  - *CRT*:_____ [RI: 1–2; <1 = compensated shock, sepsis, heat stroke; <2 = acute decompensated shock; >2 = late decompensated shock, decreased cardiac output, hypothermia]
  - *Color*:_____ [RI: pink; red = compensated shock, sepsis, heat stroke; pale/white = anemia, shock; blue = cyanosis; yellow = hepatic disease, extravascular hemolysis; brown = met-Hb]
  - *Texture*:_____ [RI: moist = hydrated; tacky-to-dry = 5–12% dehydrated]

Physical Exam – Systems Checklist:

- **Head:** _____ ☐NAF
  - Ears: ☐Ceruminous debris (mild / mod / sev) (AS / AD / AU), _____ ☐NAF
  - Eyes: _____ ☐NAF
    - ▪ Retinal: _____ ☐NAF

→ Ⓛ		Ⓡ		Ⓛ		Ⓡ ←	
☐ ⦿ Normal Direct	☐ ⦿ Normal Indirect		☐ ⦿ Normal Indirect	☐ ⦿ Normal Direct			
☐ ⦿ Abnormal Direct	☐ ⦿ Abnormal Indirect		☐ ⦿ Abnormal Indirect	☐ ⦿ Abnormal Direct			

  - Nose: _____ ☐NAF
  - Oral cavity: ☐Tarter/Gingivitis (mild / mod / sev), _____ ☐NAF
  - Mandibular lnn.: ☐Enlarged Lt., ☐Enlarged Rt., _____ ☐NAF

- **Neck:** _____ ☐NAF
  - Superficial cervical lnn.: ☐Enlarged Lt., ☐Enlarged Rt., _____ ☐NAF
  - Thyroid: _____ ☐NAF

- **Thoracic limb:** _____ ☐NAF
  - Foot pads: _____ ☐NAF
  - Knuckling: _____ ☐NAF
  - Axillary lnn. [normally absent]: _____ ☐NAF

- **Thorax:** _____ ☐NAF

- **Abdomen:** _____ ☐NAF
  - Mammary chain: _____ ☐NAF
  - Penis/ Testicles/ Vulva: _____ ☐NAF
  - Superficial inguinal lnn. [normally absent]: _____ ☐NAF

- **Pelvic limb:** _____ ☐NAF
  - Foot pads: _____ ☐NAF
  - Knuckling: _____ ☐NAF
  - Popliteal lnn.: ☐Enlarged Lt., ☐Enlarged Rt., _____ ☐NAF

- **Skin:** _____ ☐NAF
- **Tail:** _____ ☐NAF
- **Rectal☞⊙:** _____ ☐NAF

150

Problems List:

- **Problem #1**:

- **Problem #2**:

- **Problem #3**:

- **Problem #4**:

- **Problem #5**:

- **Problem #6**:

Diagnostic Plan	Treatment Plan

Case No._____

Patient	Age	Sex		Breed	Weight
		nM	sF		
	DOB:	iM	iF	Color:	kg

Owner	Primary Veterinarian	Admit Date/ Time
Name: Phone:	Name: Phone:	Date: Time: AM / PM

- **Presenting complaint**:_____
_____
_____
_____
_____
_____

- **Medical Hx**:_____
_____
_____
_____
_____
_____

- **When/ where obtained**: Date:_____; □Breeder, □Shelter, Other:_____

Drug/ Supplement	Amount	Dose (mg/kg)	Route	Frequency	Date Started

- **Vaccine status – Dog**: □Rab □Parv □Dist □Aden; □Para □Lep □Bord □Influ □Lyme
- **Vaccine status – Cat**: □Rab □Herp □Cali □Pan □FeLV [kittens]; □FIV □Chlam □Bord
- **Heartworm / Flea & Tick / Intestinal Parasites**:
  - *Last Heartworm Test*: Date:_____, □IDK; Test Results: □Pos, □Neg, □IDK
  - *Monthly heartworm preventative*: □no □yes, Product:_____
  - *Monthly flea & tick preventative*: □no □yes, Product:_____
  - *Monthly dewormer*: □no □yes, Product:_____
- **Surgical Hx**: □Spay/Neuter; Date:_____; Other:_____
- **Environment**: □Indoor, □Outdoor, Time spent outdoors/ Other:_____
- **Housemates**: Dogs:_____ Cats:_____ Other:_____
- **Diet**: □Wet, □Dry; Brand/ Amt.:_____

Appetite	□Normal, □↑, □↓
Weight	□Normal, □↑, □↓; Past Wt.:_____ kg; Date:_____; Δ:_____
Thirst	□Normal, □↑, □↓
Urination	□Normal, □↑, □↓, □Blood, □Strain
Defecation	□Normal, □↑, □↓, □Blood, □Strain, □Diarrhea, □Mucus
Discharge	□No, □Yes; Onset/ Describe:
Cough/ Sneeze	□No, □Yes; Onset/ Describe:
Vomit	□No, □Yes; Onset/ Describe:
Respiration	□Normal, □↑ Rate, □↑ Effort
Energy level	□Normal, □Lethargic, □Exercise intolerance

- **Travel Hx**: □None, Other:_____
- **Exposure to**: □Standing water, □Wildlife, □Board/daycare, □Dog park, □Groomer, □Pet store
- **Adverse reactions to food/ meds**: □None, Other:_____
- **Can give oral meds**: □no □yes; Helpful Tricks:_____

Physical Exam – General:

- **Body Weight**:_____kg   **Body Condition Score**:___/9

- **Temperature**:_____°F [*Dog-RI*: 100.9–102.4; *Cat-RI*: 98.1–102.1]

- **Heart**:
  - ○ *Rate*:_____beats/min [Dog-RI: 60–180; Cat-RI: 140–240 (in hospital)]
  - ○ *Rhythm*: ☐Regular, ☐Irregular
  - ○ *Sounds*: ☐None, ☐Split sound[S1 or S2], ☐Gallop[S3 or S4], ☐Murmur, ☐Muffled
    - ▪ *Grade*: ☐1–2[soft, only at PMI], ☐3–4[moderate, mild radiate], ☐5–6[loud, strong radiate, thrill]
    - ▪ *Timing*: ☐Systolic, ☐Diastolic, ☐Continuous
    - ▪ *PMI*:

	PMI	Over	Anatomic Boundaries
☐	Lt. apex	Mitral valve	5th to 6th ICS at level of CCJ
☐	Lt. base	Ao + Pul outflow	2nd to 4th ICS above the CCJ
☐	Rt. midheart	Tricuspid valve	3rd to 5th ICS near the CCJ
☐	Rt. sternal border	Right ventricle	5th to 7th ICS immediately dorsal to the sternum
☐	Sternal (cat)	Sternum	In cats, determination of PMI offers very little clinical significance.

   - • *Vertebral Heart Size*: Dog = 8.7–10.7; Cat = 6.9–8.1 (from cranial edge of T4)
   - • *Innocent Murmur*: Grade 1-2, systolic, left base location, disappear by ~4 months of age, absent clinical signs

- **Pulses**:
  - ○ *Pulse rate*:_____pulses/min
  - ○ *Character*: ☐Sync, ☐Async; ☐Normokinetic, ☐Hyper-, ☐Hypo-, ☐Variable

- **Lungs**:
  - ○ *Respiratory rate*:_____breaths/min [*RI*: 16–30]
  - ○ *Depth/Effort*: ☐Norm, ☐Pant, ☐Deep, ☐Shallow, ☐↑ Insp. effort, ☐↑ Exp. effort
  - ○ *Sounds/Localization*:
    - ▪ ☐Norm BV, ☐Quiet BV, ☐Loud BV, ☐Crack, ☐Wheez, ☐Frict, ☐Muffled
    - ▪ ☐All lung fields, ☐Rt cran, ☐Rt mid, ☐Rt caud, ☐Lt cran, ☐Lt mid, ☐Lt caud
  - ○ *Tracheal Auscultation/ Palpation*: ☐Normal, Other:_____

- **Pain Score**:_____ / 5   Localization:_____

- **Mentation**:

☐BAR	☐Confused/	☐Drowsy/	☐Stuporous	☐Coma
☐QAR	Disoriented	Obtunded	(unresponsive unless aroused by noxious stimuli)	(complete unresponsiveness to any stimuli)
☐Dull (conscious; responds to sensory stimuli)	(conscious; inappropriate response to environment [ex., vocalization, head pressing])	(↓ interaction with environment; slow response to verbal stimuli)		

- **Skin Elasticity**: ☐Normal skin turgor, ☐↓ Skin turgor, ☐Skin tent, ☐Gelatinous

- **Mucus Membranes**:
  - ○ *CRT*:_____ [*RI*: 1–2; <1 = compensated shock, sepsis, heat stroke; <2 = acute decompensated shock; >2 = late decompensated shock, decreased cardiac output, hypothermia]
  - ○ *Color*:_____ [*RI*: pink; red = compensated shock, sepsis, heat stroke; pale/white = anemia, shock; blue = cyanosis; yellow = hepatic disease, extravascular hemolysis; brown = met-Hb]
  - ○ *Texture*:_____ [*RI*: moist = hydrated; tacky-to-dry = 5–12% dehydrated]

Physical Exam – Systems Checklist:

- Head:_____ ☐NAF
  - Ears: ☐Ceruminous debris (mild / mod / sev) (AS / AD / AU), _____ ☐NAF
  - Eyes:_____ ☐NAF
    - Retinal:_____ ☐NAF

→ Ⓛ		Ⓡ		Ⓛ		Ⓡ ←	
☐ ⊙ Normal Direct		☐ ⊙ Normal Indirect		☐ ⊙ Normal Indirect		☐ ⊙ Normal Direct	
☐ ⦿ Abnormal Direct		☐ ⦿ Abnormal Indirect		☐ ⦿ Abnormal Indirect		☐ ⦿ Abnormal Direct	

  - Nose:_____ ☐NAF
  - Oral cavity: ☐Tarter/Gingivitis (mild / mod / sev), _____ ☐NAF
  - Mandibular lnn.: ☐Enlarged Lt., ☐Enlarged Rt., _____ ☐NAF

- Neck:_____ ☐NAF
  - Superficial cervical lnn.: ☐Enlarged Lt., ☐Enlarged Rt., _____ ☐NAF
  - Thyroid:_____ ☐NAF

- Thoracic limb:_____ ☐NAF
  - Foot pads:_____ ☐NAF
  - Knuckling:_____ ☐NAF
  - Axillary lnn. [normally absent]:_____ ☐NAF

- Thorax:_____ ☐NAF

- Abdomen:_____ ☐NAF
  - Mammary chain:_____ ☐NAF
  - Penis/ Testicles/ Vulva:_____ ☐NAF
  - Superficial inguinal lnn. [normally absent]:_____ ☐NAF

- Pelvic limb:_____ ☐NAF
  - Foot pads:_____ ☐NAF
  - Knuckling:_____ ☐NAF
  - Popliteal lnn.: ☐Enlarged Lt., ☐Enlarged Rt., _____ ☐NAF

- Skin:_____ ☐NAF
- Tail:_____ ☐NAF
- Rectal☞⊙:_____ ☐NAF

Problems List:

- **Problem #1**:

- **Problem #2**:

- **Problem #3**:

- **Problem #4**:

- **Problem #5**:

- **Problem #6**:

Diagnostic Plan	Treatment Plan

Case No._____

Patient	Age	Sex		Breed		Weight
		nM	sF			
	DOB:	iM	iF	Color:		kg

Owner		Primary Veterinarian	Admit Date/ Time
Name: Phone:		Name: Phone:	Date: Time: AM / PM

• **Presenting complaint**:_____
_____
_____
_____
_____
_____

• **Medical Hx**:_____
_____
_____
_____
_____

• **When/ where obtained**: Date:_____; □Breeder, □Shelter, Other:_____

Drug/ Supplement	Amount	Dose (mg/kg)	Route	Frequency	Date Started

• **Vaccine status – Dog**: □Rab □Parv □Dist □Aden; □Para □Lep □Bord □Influ □Lyme
• **Vaccine status – Cat**: □Rab □Herp □Cali □Pan □FeLV [kittens]; □FIV □Chlam □Bord
• **Heartworm / Flea & Tick / Intestinal Parasites**:
  ◦ *Last Heartworm Test*: Date:_____, □IDK; Test Results: □Pos, □Neg, □IDK
  ◦ *Monthly heartworm preventative*: □no □yes, Product:_____
  ◦ *Monthly flea & tick preventative*: □no □yes, Product:_____
  ◦ *Monthly dewormer*:   □no □yes, Product:_____
• **Surgical Hx**: □Spay/Neuter; Date:_____; Other:_____
• **Environment**: □Indoor, □Outdoor, Time spent outdoors/ Other:_____
• **Housemates**: Dogs:_____ Cats:_____ Other:_____
• **Diet**: □Wet, □Dry; Brand/ Amt.:_____

Appetite	□Normal, □↑, □↓
Weight	□Normal, □↑, □↓; Past Wt.:_____ kg; Date:_____; ∆:_____
Thirst	□Normal, □↑, □↓
Urination	□Normal, □↑, □↓, □Blood, □Strain
Defecation	□Normal, □↑, □↓, □Blood, □Strain, □Diarrhea, □Mucus
Discharge	□No, □Yes; Onset/ Describe:
Cough/ Sneeze	□No, □Yes; Onset/ Describe:
Vomit	□No, □Yes; Onset/ Describe:
Respiration	□Normal, □↑ Rate, □↑ Effort
Energy level	□Normal, □Lethargic, □Exercise intolerance

• **Travel Hx**: □None, Other:_____
• **Exposure to**: □Standing water, □Wildlife, □Board/daycare, □Dog park, □Groomer, □Pet store
• **Adverse reactions to food/ meds**: □None, Other:_____
• **Can give oral meds**: □no □yes; Helpful Tricks:_____

Physical Exam – General:

- **Body Weight**:_____kg **Body Condition Score**:___/9

- **Temperature**:_____°F [*Dog-RI*: 100.9–102.4; *Cat-RI*: 98.1–102.1]

- **Heart**:
  - *Rate*:_____beats/min [Dog-RI: 60–180; Cat-RI: 140–240 (in hospital)]
  - *Rhythm*: ☐Regular, ☐Irregular
  - *Sounds*: ☐None, ☐Split sound[S1 or S2], ☐Gallop[S3 or S4], ☐Murmur, ☐Muffled
    - *Grade*: ☐1–2[soft, only at PMI], ☐3–4[moderate, mild radiate], ☐5–6[loud, strong radiate, thrill]
    - *Timing*: ☐Systolic, ☐Diastolic, ☐Continuous
    - *PMI*:

	PMI	Over	Anatomic Boundaries
☐	Lt. apex	Mitral valve	5th to 6th ICS at level of CCJ
☐	Lt. base	Ao + Pul outflow	2nd to 4th ICS above the CCJ
☐	Rt. midheart	Tricuspid valve	3rd to 5th ICS near the CCJ
☐	Rt. sternal border	Right ventricle	5th to 7th ICS immediately dorsal to the sternum
☐	Sternal (cat)	Sternum	In cats, determination of PMI offers very little clinical significance.

- *Vertebral Heart Size*: Dog = 8.7–10.7; Cat = 6.9–8.1 (from cranial edge of T4)
- *Innocent Murmur*: Grade 1-2, systolic, left base location, disappear by ~4 months of age, absent clinical signs

- **Pulses**:
  - *Pulse rate*:_____pulses/min
  - *Character*: ☐Sync, ☐Async; ☐Normokinetic, ☐Hyper-, ☐Hypo-, ☐Variable

- **Lungs**:
  - *Respiratory rate*:_____breaths/min [RI: 16–30]
  - *Depth/Effort*: ☐Norm, ☐Pant, ☐Deep, ☐Shallow, ☐↑ Insp. effort, ☐↑ Exp. effort
  - *Sounds/Localization*:
    - ☐Norm BV, ☐Quiet BV, ☐Loud BV, ☐Crack, ☐Wheez, ☐Frict, ☐Muffled
    - ☐All lung fields, ☐Rt cran, ☐Rt mid, ☐Rt caud, ☐Lt cran, ☐Lt mid, ☐Lt caud
  - *Tracheal Auscultation/ Palpation*: ☐Normal, Other:_____

- **Pain Score**:_____ / 5   Localization:_____

- **Mentation**:

☐BAR ☐QAR ☐Dull (conscious; responds to sensory stimuli)	☐Confused/ Disoriented (conscious; inappropriate response to environment [ex., vocalization, head pressing])	☐Drowsy/ Obtunded (↓ interaction with environment; slow response to verbal stimuli)	☐Stuporous (unresponsive unless aroused by noxious stimuli)	☐Coma (complete unresponsiveness to any stimuli)

- **Skin Elasticity**: ☐Normal skin turgor, ☐↓ Skin turgor, ☐Skin tent, ☐Gelatinous

- **Mucus Membranes**:
  - *CRT*:_____ [RI: 1–2; <1 = compensated shock, sepsis, heat stroke; <2 = acute decompensated shock; >2 = late decompensated shock, decreased cardiac output, hypothermia]
  - *Color*:_____ [RI: pink; red = compensated shock, sepsis, heat stroke; pale/white = anemia, shock; blue = cyanosis; yellow = hepatic disease, extravascular hemolysis; brown = met-Hb]
  - *Texture*:_____ [RI: moist = hydrated; tacky-to-dry = 5–12% dehydrated]

Physical Exam – Systems Checklist:

- **Head:** _____ ☐NAF
  - Ears: ☐Ceruminous debris (mild / mod / sev) (AS / AD / AU), _____ ☐NAF
  - Eyes: _____ ☐NAF
    - Retinal: _____ ☐NAF

	→ Ⓛ		Ⓡ			Ⓛ		Ⓡ ←
☐	⊙ Normal Direct	☐	⊙ Normal Indirect		☐	⊙ Normal Indirect	☐	⊙ Normal Direct
☐	⦿ Abnormal Direct	☐	⦿ Abnormal Indirect		☐	⦿ Abnormal Indirect	☐	⦿ Abnormal Direct

  - Nose: _____ ☐NAF
  - Oral cavity: ☐Tarter/Gingivitis (mild / mod / sev), _____ ☐NAF
  - Mandibular lnn.: ☐Enlarged Lt., ☐Enlarged Rt., _____ ☐NAF

- **Neck:** _____ ☐NAF
  - Superficial cervical lnn.: ☐Enlarged Lt., ☐Enlarged Rt., _____ ☐NAF
  - Thyroid: _____ ☐NAF

- **Thoracic limb:** _____ ☐NAF
  - Foot pads: _____ ☐NAF
  - Knuckling: _____ ☐NAF
  - Axillary lnn. [normally absent]: _____ ☐NAF

- **Thorax:** _____ ☐NAF

- **Abdomen:** _____ ☐NAF
  - Mammary chain: _____ ☐NAF
  - Penis/ Testicles/ Vulva: _____ ☐NAF
  - Superficial inguinal lnn. [normally absent]: _____ ☐NAF

- **Pelvic limb:** _____ ☐NAF
  - Foot pads: _____ ☐NAF
  - Knuckling: _____ ☐NAF
  - Popliteal lnn.: ☐Enlarged Lt., ☐Enlarged Rt., _____ ☐NAF

- **Skin:** _____ ☐NAF
- **Tail:** _____ ☐NAF
- **Rectal☞⊙:** _____ ☐NAF

Problems List:

• **Problem #1**:

• **Problem #2**:

• **Problem #3**:

• **Problem #4**:

• **Problem #5**:

• **Problem #6**:

Diagnostic Plan	Treatment Plan

Case No._____

Patient	Age	Sex		Breed		Weight
		nM	sF			
	DOB:	iM	iF	Color:		kg

Owner	Primary Veterinarian	Admit Date/ Time
Name: Phone:	Name: Phone:	Date: Time: AM / PM

• Presenting complaint:_____
_____
_____
_____
_____

• Medical Hx:_____
_____
_____
_____

• When/ where obtained: Date:_____; ☐Breeder, ☐Shelter, Other:_____

Drug/ Supplement	Amount	Dose (mg/kg)	Route	Frequency	Date Started

• Vaccine status – Dog: ☐Rab ☐Parv ☐Dist ☐Aden; ☐Para ☐Lep ☐Bord ☐Influ ☐Lyme
• Vaccine status – Cat: ☐Rab ☐Herp ☐Cali ☐Pan ☐FeLV [kittens]; ☐FIV ☐Chlam ☐Bord
• Heartworm / Flea & Tick / Intestinal Parasites:
   ◦ *Last Heartworm Test*: Date:_____, ☐IDK; Test Results: ☐Pos, ☐Neg, ☐IDK
   ◦ *Monthly heartworm preventative*: ☐no ☐yes, Product:_____
   ◦ *Monthly flea & tick preventative*: ☐no ☐yes, Product:_____
   ◦ *Monthly dewormer*:   ☐no ☐yes, Product:_____
• Surgical Hx: ☐Spay/Neuter; Date:_____; Other:_____
• Environment: ☐Indoor, ☐Outdoor, Time spent outdoors/ Other:_____
• Housemates: Dogs:_____ Cats:_____ Other:_____
• Diet: ☐Wet, ☐Dry; Brand/ Amt.:_____

Appetite	☐Normal, ☐↑, ☐↓
Weight	☐Normal, ☐↑, ☐↓; Past Wt.:_____ kg; Date:_____; Δ:_____
Thirst	☐Normal, ☐↑, ☐↓
Urination	☐Normal, ☐↑, ☐↓, ☐Blood, ☐Strain
Defecation	☐Normal, ☐↑, ☐↓, ☐Blood, ☐Strain, ☐Diarrhea, ☐Mucus
Discharge	☐No, ☐Yes; Onset/ Describe:
Cough/ Sneeze	☐No, ☐Yes; Onset/ Describe:
Vomit	☐No, ☐Yes; Onset/ Describe:
Respiration	☐Normal, ☐↑ Rate, ☐↑ Effort
Energy level	☐Normal, ☐Lethargic, ☐Exercise intolerance

• Travel Hx: ☐None, Other:_____
• Exposure to: ☐Standing water, ☐Wildlife, ☐Board/daycare, ☐Dog park, ☐Groomer, ☐Pet store
• Adverse reactions to food/ meds: ☐None, Other:_____
• Can give oral meds: ☐no ☐yes; Helpful Tricks:_____

Physical Exam – General:

- **Body Weight**:_____kg   **Body Condition Score**:____/9

- **Temperature**:_____°F [*Dog-RI*: 100.9–102.4; *Cat-RI*: 98.1–102.1]

- **Heart**:
  - *Rate*:_____beats/min [Dog-RI: 60–180; Cat-RI: 140–240 (in hospital)]
  - *Rhythm*: ☐Regular, ☐Irregular
  - *Sounds*: ☐None, ☐Split sound[S1 or S2], ☐Gallop[S3 or S4], ☐Murmur, ☐Muffled
    - *Grade*: ☐1–2[soft, only at PMI], ☐3–4[moderate, mild radiate], ☐5–6[loud, strong radiate, thrill]
    - *Timing*: ☐Systolic, ☐Diastolic, ☐Continuous
    - *PMI*:

	PMI	Over	Anatomic Boundaries
☐	Lt. apex	Mitral valve	5th to 6th ICS at level of CCJ
☐	Lt. base	Ao + Pul outflow	2nd to 4th ICS above the CCJ
☐	Rt. midheart	Tricuspid valve	3rd to 5th ICS near the CCJ
☐	Rt. sternal border	Right ventricle	5th to 7th ICS immediately dorsal to the sternum
☐	Sternal (cat)	Sternum	In cats, determination of PMI offers very little clinical significance.

  - *Vertebral Heart Size*: Dog = 8.7–10.7; Cat = 6.9–8.1 (from cranial edge of T4)
  - *Innocent Murmur*: Grade 1-2, systolic, left base location, disappear by ~4 months of age, absent clinical signs

- **Pulses**:
  - *Pulse rate*:_____pulses/min
  - *Character*: ☐Sync, ☐Async; ☐Normokinetic, ☐Hyper-, ☐Hypo-, ☐Variable

- **Lungs**:
  - *Respiratory rate*:_____breaths/min [*RI*: 16–30]
  - *Depth/Effort*: ☐Norm, ☐Pant, ☐Deep, ☐Shallow, ☐↑ Insp. effort, ☐↑ Exp. effort
  - *Sounds/Localization*:
    - ☐Norm BV, ☐Quiet BV, ☐Loud BV, ☐Crack, ☐Wheez, ☐Frict, ☐Muffled
    - ☐All lung fields, ☐Rt cran, ☐Rt mid, ☐Rt caud, ☐Lt cran, ☐Lt mid, ☐Lt caud
  - *Tracheal Auscultation/ Palpation*: ☐Normal, Other:_____

- **Pain Score**:_____ / 5   Localization:_____

- **Mentation**: ☐BAR   ☐Confused/   ☐Drowsy/   ☐Stuporous   ☐Coma
  ☐QAR   Disoriented   Obtunded   (unresponsive unless   (complete
  ☐Dull   (conscious; inappropriate (↓ interaction with   aroused by noxious   unresponsiveness
  (conscious; responds   response to environment environment; slow   stimuli)   to any stimuli)
  to sensory stimuli)   [ex., vocalization, head response to verbal
                         pressing])   stimuli)

- **Skin Elasticity**: ☐Normal skin turgor, ☐↓ Skin turgor, ☐Skin tent, ☐Gelatinous

- **Mucus Membranes**:
  - *CRT*:_____ [*RI*: 1–2; <1 = compensated shock, sepsis, heat stroke; <2 = acute decompensated shock; >2 = late decompensated shock, decreased cardiac output, hypothermia]
  - *Color*:_____ [*RI*: pink; red = compensated shock, sepsis, heat stroke; pale/white = anemia, shock; blue = cyanosis; yellow = hepatic disease, extravascular hemolysis; brown = met-Hb]
  - *Texture*:_____ [*RI*: moist = hydrated; tacky-to-dry = 5–12% dehydrated]

Physical Exam – Systems Checklist:

- Head: _____ ☐NAF
  - Ears: ☐Ceruminous debris (mild / mod / sev) (AS / AD / AU), _____ ☐NAF
  - Eyes: _____ ☐NAF
    - Retinal: _____ ☐NAF

→ ⓛ		ⓡ		ⓛ		ⓡ ←	
☐ ⊙ Normal Direct	☐ ⊙ Normal Indirect	☐ ⊙ Normal Indirect	☐ ⊙ Normal Direct
☐ ⦿ Abnormal Direct	☐ ⦿ Abnormal Indirect	☐ ⦿ Abnormal Indirect	☐ ⦿ Abnormal Direct

  - Nose: _____ ☐NAF
  - Oral cavity: ☐Tarter/Gingivitis (mild / mod / sev), _____ ☐NAF
  - Mandibular lnn.: ☐Enlarged Lt., ☐Enlarged Rt., _____ ☐NAF

- Neck: _____ ☐NAF
  - Superficial cervical lnn.: ☐Enlarged Lt., ☐Enlarged Rt., _____ ☐NAF
  - Thyroid: _____ ☐NAF

- Thoracic limb: _____ ☐NAF
  - Foot pads: _____ ☐NAF
  - Knuckling: _____ ☐NAF
  - Axillary lnn. [normally absent]: _____ ☐NAF

- Thorax: _____ ☐NAF

- Abdomen: _____ ☐NAF
  - Mammary chain: _____ ☐NAF
  - Penis/ Testicles/ Vulva: _____ ☐NAF
  - Superficial inguinal lnn. [normally absent]: _____ ☐NAF

- Pelvic limb: _____ ☐NAF
  - Foot pads: _____ ☐NAF
  - Knuckling: _____ ☐NAF
  - Popliteal lnn.: ☐Enlarged Lt., ☐Enlarged Rt., _____ ☐NAF

- Skin: _____ ☐NAF
- Tail: _____ ☐NAF
- Rectal☞☉: _____ ☐NAF

Problems List:

• **Problem #1**:

• **Problem #2**:

• **Problem #3**:

• **Problem #4**:

• **Problem #5**:

• **Problem #6**:

Diagnostic Plan	Treatment Plan

Case No._____

Patient	Age	Sex		Breed	Weight
		nM	sF		kg
	DOB:	iM	iF	Color:	

Owner	Primary Veterinarian	Admit Date/ Time
Name: Phone:	Name: Phone:	Date: Time: AM / PM

• **Presenting complaint**:_____
_____
_____
_____
_____
_____

• **Medical Hx**:_____
_____
_____
_____
_____

• **When/ where obtained**: Date:_____; □Breeder, □Shelter, Other:_____

Drug/ Supplement	Amount	Dose (mg/kg)	Route	Frequency	Date Started

• **Vaccine status – Dog**: □Rab □Parv □Dist □Aden; □Para □Lep □Bord □Influ □Lyme
• **Vaccine status – Cat**: □Rab □Herp □Cali □Pan □FeLV [kittens]; □FIV □Chlam □Bord
• **Heartworm / Flea & Tick / Intestinal Parasites**:
  ◦ *Last Heartworm Test*: Date:_____, □IDK; Test Results: □Pos, □Neg, □IDK
  ◦ *Monthly heartworm preventative*: □no □yes, Product:_____
  ◦ *Monthly flea & tick preventative*: □no □yes, Product:_____
  ◦ *Monthly dewormer*:   □no □yes, Product:_____
• **Surgical Hx**: □Spay/Neuter; Date:_____; Other:_____
• **Environment**: □Indoor, □Outdoor, Time spent outdoors/ Other:_____
• **Housemates**: Dogs:_____ Cats:_____ Other:_____
• **Diet**: □Wet, □Dry; Brand/ Amt.:_____

Appetite	□Normal, □↑, □↓
Weight	□Normal, □↑, □↓; Past Wt.:_____ kg; Date:_____; Δ:_____
Thirst	□Normal, □↑, □↓
Urination	□Normal, □↑, □↓, □Blood, □Strain
Defecation	□Normal, □↑, □↓, □Blood, □Strain, □Diarrhea, □Mucus
Discharge	□No, □Yes; Onset/ Describe:
Cough/ Sneeze	□No, □Yes; Onset/ Describe:
Vomit	□No, □Yes; Onset/ Describe:
Respiration	□Normal, □↑ Rate, □↑ Effort
Energy level	□Normal, □Lethargic, □Exercise intolerance

• **Travel Hx**: □None, Other:_____
• **Exposure to**: □Standing water, □Wildlife, □Board/daycare, □Dog park, □Groomer, □Pet store
• **Adverse reactions to food/ meds**: □None, Other:_____
• **Can give oral meds**: □no □yes; Helpful Tricks:_____

Physical Exam – General:

- **Body Weight**:_____kg　　**Body Condition Score**:___/9

- **Temperature**:_____°F [*Dog-RI*: 100.9–102.4;　*Cat-RI*: 98.1–102.1]

- **Heart**:
  - *Rate*:_____beats/min [Dog-RI: 60–180;　Cat-RI: 140–240 (in hospital)]
  - *Rhythm*: ☐Regular, ☐Irregular
  - *Sounds*: ☐None, ☐Split sound[S1 or S2], ☐Gallop[S3 or S4], ☐Murmur, ☐Muffled
    - *Grade*: ☐1–2[soft, only at PMI], ☐3–4[moderate, mild radiate], ☐5–6[loud, strong radiate, thrill]
    - *Timing*: ☐Systolic, ☐Diastolic, ☐Continuous
    - *PMI*:

	PMI	Over	Anatomic Boundaries
☐	Lt. apex	Mitral valve	5th to 6th ICS at level of CCJ
☐	Lt. base	Ao + Pul outflow	2nd to 4th ICS above the CCJ
☐	Rt. midheart	Tricuspid valve	3rd to 5th ICS near the CCJ
☐	Rt. sternal border	Right ventricle	5th to 7th ICS immediately dorsal to the sternum
☐	Sternal (cat)	Sternum	In cats, determination of PMI offers very little clinical significance.

- *Vertebral Heart Size*: Dog = 8.7–10.7; Cat = 6.9–8.1 (from cranial edge of T4)
- *Innocent Murmur*: Grade 1-2, systolic, left base location, disappear by ~4 months of age, absent clinical signs

- **Pulses**:
  - *Pulse rate*:_____pulses/min
  - *Character*: ☐Sync, ☐Async;　☐Normokinetic, ☐Hyper-, ☐Hypo-, ☐Variable

- **Lungs**:
  - *Respiratory rate*:_____breaths/min [RI: 16–30]
  - *Depth/Effort*: ☐Norm, ☐Pant, ☐Deep, ☐Shallow, ☐↑ Insp. effort, ☐↑ Exp. effort
  - *Sounds/Localization*:
    - ☐Norm BV, ☐Quiet BV, ☐Loud BV, ☐Crack, ☐Wheez, ☐Frict, ☐Muffled
    - ☐All lung fields, ☐Rt cran, ☐Rt mid, ☐Rt caud, ☐Lt cran, ☐Lt mid, ☐Lt caud
  - *Tracheal Auscultation/ Palpation*: ☐Normal, Other:_____

- **Pain Score**:_____ / 5　Localization:_____

- **Mentation**:

☐BAR	☐Confused/	☐Drowsy/	☐Stuporous	☐Coma
☐QAR	Disoriented	Obtunded	(unresponsive unless aroused by noxious stimuli)	(complete unresponsiveness to any stimuli)
☐Dull (conscious; responds to sensory stimuli)	(conscious; inappropriate response to environment [ex., vocalization, head pressing])	(↓ interaction with environment; slow response to verbal stimuli)		

- **Skin Elasticity**: ☐Normal skin turgor, ☐↓ Skin turgor, ☐Skin tent, ☐Gelatinous

- **Mucus Membranes**:
  - *CRT*:_____ [RI: 1–2; <1 = compensated shock, sepsis, heat stroke; <2 = acute decompensated shock; >2 = late decompensated shock, decreased cardiac output, hypothermia]
  - *Color*:_____ [RI: pink; red = compensated shock, sepsis, heat stroke; pale/white = anemia, shock; blue = cyanosis; yellow = hepatic disease, extravascular hemolysis; brown = met-Hb]
  - *Texture*:_____ [RI: moist = hydrated; tacky-to-dry = 5–12% dehydrated]

Physical Exam – Systems Checklist:

- Head:_____ ☐NAF
  - Ears: ☐Ceruminous debris (mild / mod / sev) (AS / AD / AU),_____ ☐NAF
  - Eyes:_____ ☐NAF
    - Retinal:_____ ☐NAF

→ Ⓛ		Ⓡ		Ⓛ		Ⓡ ←	
☐ ⊙ Normal Direct	☐ ⊙ Normal Indirect	☐ ⊙ Normal Indirect	☐ ⊙ Normal Direct
☐ ⬤ Abnormal Direct	☐ ⬤ Abnormal Indirect	☐ ⬤ Abnormal Indirect	☐ ⬤ Abnormal Direct

  - Nose:_____ ☐NAF
  - Oral cavity: ☐Tarter/Gingivitis (mild / mod / sev),_____ ☐NAF
  - Mandibular lnn.: ☐Enlarged Lt., ☐Enlarged Rt.,_____ ☐NAF

- Neck:_____ ☐NAF
  - Superficial cervical lnn.: ☐Enlarged Lt., ☐Enlarged Rt.,_____ ☐NAF
  - Thyroid:_____ ☐NAF

- Thoracic limb:_____ ☐NAF
  - Foot pads:_____ ☐NAF
  - Knuckling:_____ ☐NAF
  - Axillary lnn. [normally absent]:_____ ☐NAF

- Thorax:_____ ☐NAF

- Abdomen:_____ ☐NAF
  - Mammary chain:_____ ☐NAF
  - Penis/ Testicles/ Vulva:_____ ☐NAF
  - Superficial inguinal lnn. [normally absent]:_____ ☐NAF

- Pelvic limb:_____ ☐NAF
  - Foot pads:_____ ☐NAF
  - Knuckling:_____ ☐NAF
  - Popliteal lnn.: ☐Enlarged Lt., ☐Enlarged Rt.,_____ ☐NAF

- Skin:_____ ☐NAF
- Tail:_____ ☐NAF
- Rectal☞☉:_____ ☐NAF

Problems List:

• **Problem #1**:

• **Problem #2**:

• **Problem #3**:

• **Problem #4**:

• **Problem #5**:

• **Problem #6**:

Diagnostic Plan	Treatment Plan

Case No._____

Patient	Age	Sex		Breed	Weight
		nM	sF		
	DOB:	iM	iF	Color:	kg

Owner	Primary Veterinarian	Admit Date/ Time
Name: Phone:	Name: Phone:	Date: Time: AM / PM

• **Presenting complaint**:_____
_____
_____
_____
_____

• **Medical Hx**:_____
_____
_____
_____
_____

• **When/ where obtained**: Date:_____; ☐Breeder, ☐Shelter, Other:_____

Drug/ Supplement	Amount	Dose (mg/kg)	Route	Frequency	Date Started

• **Vaccine status – Dog**: ☐Rab ☐Parv ☐Dist ☐Aden; ☐Para ☐Lep ☐Bord ☐Influ ☐Lyme
• **Vaccine status – Cat**: ☐Rab ☐Herp ☐Cali ☐Pan ☐FeLV [kittens]; ☐FIV ☐Chlam ☐Bord
• **Heartworm / Flea & Tick / Intestinal Parasites**:
  ◦ *Last Heartworm Test*: Date:_____, ☐IDK; Test Results: ☐Pos, ☐Neg, ☐IDK
  ◦ *Monthly heartworm preventative*: ☐no ☐yes, Product:_____
  ◦ *Monthly flea & tick preventative*: ☐no ☐yes, Product:_____
  ◦ *Monthly dewormer*: ☐no ☐yes, Product:_____
• **Surgical Hx**: ☐Spay/Neuter; Date:_____; Other:_____
• **Environment**: ☐Indoor, ☐Outdoor, Time spent outdoors/ Other:_____
• **Housemates**: Dogs:_____ Cats:_____ Other:_____
• **Diet**: ☐Wet, ☐Dry; Brand/ Amt.:_____

Appetite	☐Normal, ☐↑, ☐↓
Weight	☐Normal, ☐↑, ☐↓; Past Wt.:_____ kg; Date:_____; Δ:_____
Thirst	☐Normal, ☐↑, ☐↓
Urination	☐Normal, ☐↑, ☐↓, ☐Blood, ☐Strain
Defecation	☐Normal, ☐↑, ☐↓, ☐Blood, ☐Strain, ☐Diarrhea, ☐Mucus
Discharge	☐No, ☐Yes; Onset/ Describe:
Cough/ Sneeze	☐No, ☐Yes; Onset/ Describe:
Vomit	☐No, ☐Yes; Onset/ Describe:
Respiration	☐Normal, ☐↑ Rate, ☐↑ Effort
Energy level	☐Normal, ☐Lethargic, ☐Exercise intolerance

• **Travel Hx**: ☐None, Other:_____
• **Exposure to**: ☐Standing water, ☐Wildlife, ☐Board/daycare, ☐Dog park, ☐Groomer, ☐Pet store
• **Adverse reactions to food/ meds**: ☐None, Other:_____
• **Can give oral meds**: ☐no ☐yes; Helpful Tricks:_____

Physical Exam – General:

- **Body Weight:**_____kg   **Body Condition Score:**___/9

- **Temperature:**_____°F [*Dog-RI*: 100.9–102.4; *Cat-RI*: 98.1–102.1]

- **Heart:**
  - *Rate:*_____beats/min [Dog-RI: 60–180; Cat-RI: 140–240 (in hospital)]
  - *Rhythm:* ☐Regular, ☐Irregular
  - *Sounds:* ☐None, ☐Split sound[S1 or S2], ☐Gallop[S3 or S4], ☐Murmur, ☐Muffled
    - *Grade:* ☐1–2[soft, only at PMI], ☐3–4[moderate, mild radiate], ☐5–6[loud, strong radiate, thrill]
    - *Timing:* ☐Systolic, ☐Diastolic, ☐Continuous
    - *PMI:*

	PMI	Over	Anatomic Boundaries
☐	Lt. apex	Mitral valve	5th to 6th ICS at level of CCJ
☐	Lt. base	Ao + Pul outflow	2nd to 4th ICS above the CCJ
☐	Rt. midheart	Tricuspid valve	3rd to 5th ICS near the CCJ
☐	Rt. sternal border	Right ventricle	5th to 7th ICS immediately dorsal to the sternum
☐	Sternal (cat)	Sternum	In cats, determination of PMI offers very little clinical significance.

  - *Vertebral Heart Size:* Dog = 8.7–10.7; Cat = 6.9–8.1 (from cranial edge of T4)
  - *Innocent Murmur:* Grade 1-2, systolic, left base location, disappear by ~4 months of age, absent clinical signs

- **Pulses:**
  - *Pulse rate:*_____pulses/min
  - *Character:* ☐Sync, ☐Async;   ☐Normokinetic, ☐Hyper-, ☐Hypo-, ☐Variable

- **Lungs:**
  - *Respiratory rate:*_____breaths/min [*RI*: 16–30]
  - *Depth/Effort:* ☐Norm, ☐Pant, ☐Deep, ☐Shallow, ☐↑ Insp. effort, ☐↑ Exp. effort
  - *Sounds/Localization:*
    - ☐Norm BV, ☐Quiet BV, ☐Loud BV, ☐Crack, ☐Wheez, ☐Frict, ☐Muffled
    - ☐All lung fields, ☐Rt cran, ☐Rt mid, ☐Rt caud, ☐Lt cran, ☐Lt mid, ☐Lt caud
  - *Tracheal Auscultation/ Palpation:* ☐Normal, Other:_____

- **Pain Score:**_____/ 5   Localization:_____

- **Mentation:**

☐BAR	☐Confused/	☐Drowsy/	☐Stuporous	☐Coma
☐QAR	Disoriented	Obtunded	(unresponsive unless aroused by noxious stimuli)	(complete unresponsiveness to any stimuli)
☐Dull (conscious; responds to sensory stimuli)	(conscious; inappropriate response to environment [ex., vocalization, head pressing])	(↓ interaction with environment; slow response to verbal stimuli)		

- **Skin Elasticity:** ☐Normal skin turgor, ☐↓ Skin turgor, ☐Skin tent, ☐Gelatinous

- **Mucus Membranes:**
  - *CRT:*_____ [*RI*: 1–2; <1 = compensated shock, sepsis, heat stroke; <2 = acute decompensated shock; >2 = late decompensated shock, decreased cardiac output, hypothermia]
  - *Color:*_____ [*RI*: pink; red = compensated shock, sepsis, heat stroke; pale/white = anemia, shock; blue = cyanosis; yellow = hepatic disease, extravascular hemolysis; brown = met-Hb]
  - *Texture:*_____ [*RI*: moist = hydrated; tacky-to-dry = 5–12% dehydrated]

Physical Exam – Systems Checklist:

- Head:_____ ☐NAF
  - Ears: ☐Ceruminous debris (mild / mod / sev) (AS / AD / AU), _____ ☐NAF
  - Eyes:_____ ☐NAF
    - Retinal:_____ ☐NAF

→ Ⓛ		Ⓡ		Ⓛ		Ⓡ ←	
☐ ⊙ Normal Direct	☐ ⊙ Normal Indirect	☐ ⊙ Normal Indirect	☐ ⊙ Normal Direct
☐ ⊙ Abnormal Direct	☐ ⊙ Abnormal Indirect	☐ ⊙ Abnormal Indirect	☐ ⊙ Abnormal Direct

  - Nose:_____ ☐NAF
  - Oral cavity: ☐Tarter/Gingivitis (mild / mod / sev), _____ ☐NAF
  - Mandibular lnn.: ☐Enlarged Lt., ☐Enlarged Rt., _____ ☐NAF

- Neck:_____ ☐NAF
  - Superficial cervical lnn.: ☐Enlarged Lt., ☐Enlarged Rt., _____ ☐NAF
  - Thyroid:_____ ☐NAF

- Thoracic limb:_____ ☐NAF
  - Foot pads:_____ ☐NAF
  - Knuckling:_____ ☐NAF
  - Axillary lnn. [normally absent]:_____ ☐NAF

- Thorax:_____ ☐NAF

- Abdomen:_____ ☐NAF
  - Mammary chain:_____ ☐NAF
  - Penis/ Testicles/ Vulva:_____ ☐NAF
  - Superficial inguinal lnn. [normally absent]:_____ ☐NAF

- Pelvic limb:_____ ☐NAF
  - Foot pads:_____ ☐NAF
  - Knuckling:_____ ☐NAF
  - Popliteal lnn.: ☐Enlarged Lt., ☐Enlarged Rt., _____ ☐NAF

- Skin:_____ ☐NAF
- Tail:_____ ☐NAF
- Rectal☞⊙:_____ ☐NAF

Problems List:

- **Problem #1**:

- **Problem #2**:

- **Problem #3**:

- **Problem #4**:

- **Problem #5**:

- **Problem #6**:

Diagnostic Plan	Treatment Plan

Case No._____

Patient	Age	Sex		Breed	Weight
		nM	sF		
	DOB:	iM	iF	Color:	kg

Owner	Primary Veterinarian	Admit Date/ Time
Name: Phone:	Name: Phone:	Date: Time: AM / PM

• **Presenting complaint**:_____
_____
_____
_____
_____

• **Medical Hx**:_____
_____
_____
_____

• **When/ where obtained**: Date:_____; □Breeder, □Shelter, Other:_____

Drug/ Supplement	Amount	Dose (mg/kg)	Route	Frequency	Date Started

• **Vaccine status – Dog**: □Rab □Parv □Dist □Aden; □Para □Lep □Bord □Influ □Lyme
• **Vaccine status – Cat**: □Rab □Herp □Cali □Pan □FeLV [kittens]; □FIV □Chlam □Bord
• **Heartworm / Flea & Tick / Intestinal Parasites**:
  ◦ *Last Heartworm Test*: Date:_____, □IDK; Test Results: □Pos, □Neg, □IDK
  ◦ *Monthly heartworm preventative*: □no □yes, Product:_____
  ◦ *Monthly flea & tick preventative*: □no □yes, Product:_____
  ◦ *Monthly dewormer*:   □no □yes, Product:_____
• **Surgical Hx**: □Spay/Neuter; Date:_____; Other:_____
• **Environment**: □Indoor, □Outdoor, Time spent outdoors/ Other:_____
• **Housemates**: Dogs:____ Cats:____ Other:_____
• **Diet**: □Wet, □Dry; Brand/ Amt.:_____

Appetite	□Normal, □↑, □↓
Weight	□Normal, □↑, □↓; Past Wt.:_____ kg; Date:_____; Δ:_____
Thirst	□Normal, □↑, □↓
Urination	□Normal, □↑, □↓, □Blood, □Strain
Defecation	□Normal, □↑, □↓, □Blood, □Strain, □Diarrhea, □Mucus
Discharge	□No, □Yes; Onset/ Describe:
Cough/ Sneeze	□No, □Yes; Onset/ Describe:
Vomit	□No, □Yes; Onset/ Describe:
Respiration	□Normal, □↑ Rate, □↑ Effort
Energy level	□Normal, □Lethargic, □Exercise intolerance

• **Travel Hx**: □None, Other:_____
• **Exposure to**: □Standing water, □Wildlife, □Board/daycare, □Dog park, □Groomer, □Pet store
• **Adverse reactions to food/ meds**: □None, Other:_____
• **Can give oral meds**: □no □yes; Helpful Tricks:_____

Physical Exam – General:

- **Body Weight:**_____ kg   **Body Condition Score:**____/9

- **Temperature:**_____°F [*Dog-RI*: 100.9–102.4; *Cat-RI*: 98.1–102.1]

- **Heart:**
  - *Rate:*_____ beats/min [Dog-RI: 60–180; Cat-RI: 140–240 (in hospital)]
  - *Rhythm:* ☐Regular, ☐Irregular
  - *Sounds:* ☐None, ☐Split sound[S1 or S2], ☐Gallop[S3 or S4], ☐Murmur, ☐Muffled
    - *Grade:* ☐1–2[soft, only at PMI], ☐3–4[moderate, mild radiate], ☐5–6[loud, strong radiate, thrill]
    - *Timing:* ☐Systolic, ☐Diastolic, ☐Continuous
    - *PMI:*

	PMI	Over	Anatomic Boundaries
☐	Lt. apex	Mitral valve	5th to 6th ICS at level of CCJ
☐	Lt. base	Ao + Pul outflow	2nd to 4th ICS above the CCJ
☐	Rt. midheart	Tricuspid valve	3rd to 5th ICS near the CCJ
☐	Rt. sternal border	Right ventricle	5th to 7th ICS immediately dorsal to the sternum
☐	Sternal (cat)	Sternum	In cats, determination of PMI offers very little clinical significance.

  - *Vertebral Heart Size*: Dog = 8.7–10.7; Cat = 6.9–8.1 (from cranial edge of T4)
  - *Innocent Murmur*: Grade 1-2, systolic, left base location, disappear by ~4 months of age, absent clinical signs

- **Pulses:**
  - *Pulse rate:*_____ pulses/min
  - *Character:* ☐Sync, ☐Async; ☐Normokinetic, ☐Hyper-, ☐Hypo-, ☐Variable

- **Lungs:**
  - *Respiratory rate:*_____ breaths/min [*RI*: 16–30]
  - *Depth/Effort:* ☐Norm, ☐Pant, ☐Deep, ☐Shallow, ☐↑ Insp. effort, ☐↑ Exp. effort
  - *Sounds/Localization:*
    - ☐Norm BV, ☐Quiet BV, ☐Loud BV, ☐Crack, ☐Wheez, ☐Frict, ☐Muffled
    - ☐All lung fields, ☐Rt cran, ☐Rt mid, ☐Rt caud, ☐Lt cran, ☐Lt mid, ☐Lt caud
  - *Tracheal Auscultation/ Palpation:* ☐Normal, Other:_____

- **Pain Score:**_____ / 5   Localization:_____

- **Mentation:** ☐BAR ☐Confused/ ☐Drowsy/ ☐Stuporous ☐Coma

☐BAR ☐QAR ☐Dull (conscious; responds to sensory stimuli)	☐Confused/ Disoriented (conscious; inappropriate response to environment [ex., vocalization, head pressing])	☐Drowsy/ Obtunded (↓ interaction with environment; slow response to verbal stimuli)	☐Stuporous (unresponsive unless aroused by noxious stimuli)	☐Coma (complete unresponsiveness to any stimuli)

- **Skin Elasticity:** ☐Normal skin turgor, ☐↓ Skin turgor, ☐Skin tent, ☐Gelatinous

- **Mucus Membranes:**
  - *CRT:*_____ [*RI*: 1–2; <1 = compensated shock, sepsis, heat stroke; <2 = acute decompensated shock; >2 = late decompensated shock, decreased cardiac output, hypothermia]
  - *Color:*_____ [*RI*: pink; red = compensated shock, sepsis, heat stroke; pale/white = anemia, shock; blue = cyanosis; yellow = hepatic disease, extravascular hemolysis; brown = met-Hb]
  - *Texture:*_____ [*RI*: moist = hydrated; tacky-to-dry = 5–12% dehydrated]

Physical Exam – Systems Checklist:

- Head:_____ ☐NAF
  - Ears: ☐Ceruminous debris (mild / mod / sev) (AS / AD / AU), _____ ☐NAF
  - Eyes:_____ ☐NAF
    - Retinal:_____ ☐NAF

→ Ⓛ		Ⓡ		Ⓛ		Ⓡ ←	
☐	⊙ Normal Direct	☐	⊙ Normal Indirect	☐	⊙ Normal Indirect	☐	⊙ Normal Direct
☐	● Abnormal Direct	☐	● Abnormal Indirect	☐	● Abnormal Indirect	☐	● Abnormal Direct

  - Nose:_____ ☐NAF
  - Oral cavity: ☐Tarter/Gingivitis (mild / mod / sev), _____ ☐NAF
  - Mandibular lnn.: ☐Enlarged Lt., ☐Enlarged Rt., _____ ☐NAF

- Neck:_____ ☐NAF
  - Superficial cervical lnn.: ☐Enlarged Lt., ☐Enlarged Rt., _____ ☐NAF
  - Thyroid:_____ ☐NAF

- Thoracic limb:_____ ☐NAF
  - Foot pads:_____ ☐NAF
  - Knuckling:_____ ☐NAF
  - Axillary lnn. [normally absent]:_____ ☐NAF

- Thorax:_____ ☐NAF

- Abdomen:_____ ☐NAF
  - Mammary chain:_____ ☐NAF
  - Penis/ Testicles/ Vulva:_____ ☐NAF
  - Superficial inguinal lnn. [normally absent]:_____ ☐NAF

- Pelvic limb:_____ ☐NAF
  - Foot pads:_____ ☐NAF
  - Knuckling:_____ ☐NAF
  - Popliteal lnn.: ☐Enlarged Lt., ☐Enlarged Rt., _____ ☐NAF

- Skin:_____ ☐NAF
- Tail:_____ ☐NAF
- Rectal☞☉:_____ ☐NAF

Problems List:

• **Problem #1**:

• **Problem #2**:

• **Problem #3**:

• **Problem #4**:

• **Problem #5**:

• **Problem #6**:

Diagnostic Plan	Treatment Plan

[Intentionally Left Blank]

Orthopedic, Neurologic, and Optic Exams

Orthopedic Examination:

- **Patient**:_____

- **Date**:_____

- General Appearance:
    - ○ Disposition:_____
    - ○ Weight status:_____
    - ○ Limb alignment:_____
    - ○ Positive (failed) sit test: ☐yes, ☐no _____
    - ○ Overt:
        - ▪ Lameness: _____ ☐NAF
        - ▪ Asym. joint swellings:_____ ☐NAF
        - ▪ Asym. soft tis. Swellings:_____ ☐NAF
        - ▪ Muscle atrophy:_____ ☐NAF

- Gait evaluation:
    [*Abnormality examples*: shortened stride, dragging of the toe-nails, toeing-in or toeing-out, limb circumduction, long-strided gait, meniscal click, head bob, *stumbling, *ataxia, *tetraparesis, or *paraparesis (*findings that suggest neuro)]
    - ○ Abnormalities at walk: ☐None, Other:_____
    - ○ Abnormalities at trot: ☐None, Other:_____

- Standing Palpation:
    [*Abnormality examples*: jt. effusion or thickening (medial buttress), heat, malalignment of bony landmarks, crepitus, atrophy]
    - ○ *Thoracic Limb*:
        - ▪ Acromion:_____ ☐NAF
        - ▪ Spine of scapula:_____ ☐NAF
        - ▪ G. tubercle of hum.:_____ ☐NAF
        - ▪ Hum. epicondyles:_____ ☐NAF
        - ▪ Olecranon:_____ ☐NAF
        - ▪ Acc. carpal bn.:_____ ☐NAF
        - ▪ Conscious proprioception:_____ ☐NAF

    - ○ *Pelvic Limb*:
        - ▪ Normal triangular orientation of ilial wing, tuber ischii, and greater trochanter:
          ☐yes, ☐no [Linear orientation of landmarks indicates craniodorsal hip luxation.]
        - ▪ Iliac crest:_____ ☐NAF
        - ▪ Ischiatic tuberosity:_____ ☐NAF
        - ▪ G. trochanter of fem.:_____ ☐NAF
        - ▪ Quadriceps m.:_____ ☐NAF
        - ▪ Patella/ patellar ten.:_____ ☐NAF
            - • Able to define cranial 2/3 of patellar tendon: ☐yes, ☐no _____
            - • Patellar luxation: ☐yes, ☐no _____
                - ☐1(In-Out-In), ☐2(In-Out-Out), ☐3(Out-In-Out), ☐4(Out-Out-Out)
        - ▪ Tibial tuberosity:_____ ☐NAF
        - ▪ Hamstring mm.:_____ ☐NAF
        - ▪ Femoral condyles:_____ ☐NAF
        - ▪ Distal tibia:_____ ☐NAF
        - ▪ Achilles tendon:_____ ☐NAF
        - ▪ Tuber calcaneous:_____ ☐NAF
        - ▪ Tarsal joint:_____ ☐NAF
        - ▪ Conscious proprioception:_____ ☐NAF

    - ○ *Vertebral Column*:
        - ▪ Spinal hyperesthesia: ☐yes, ☐no _____
        - ▪ Tail pain: ☐yes, ☐no _____
        - ▪ Sacroiliac jt. pain: ☐yes, ☐no _____

- <u>Recumbent Palpation:</u>
  - *[Abnormality examples: CREPI – crepitus, decreased range-of-motion, effusion, pain, instability]*
    - ○ *Right Thoracic Limb:*
      - Footpads/ interdigital webs:_____ ☐NAF
      - Flex/ extend digital joints:_____ ☐NAF
      - Flex/ extend/ varus/ valgus of carpal joints:_____ ☐NAF
      - Flex/ extend elbow joint:_____ ☐NAF
      - Int./ ext. rotation of elbow w/ med. digital pres.:_____ ☐NAF
      - Flex/ extend shoulder joint:_____ ☐NAF

    - ○ *Left Thoracic Limb:*
      - Footpads/ interdigital webs:_____ ☐NAF
      - Flex/ extend digital joints:_____ ☐NAF
      - Flex/ extend/ varus/ valgus of carpal joints:_____ ☐NAF
      - Flex/ extend elbow joint:_____ ☐NAF
      - Int./ ext. rotation of elbow w/ med. digital pres.:_____ ☐NAF
      - Flex/ extend shoulder joint:_____ ☐NAF

    - ○ *Right Pelvic Limb:*
      - Footpads/ interdigital webs:_____ ☐NAF
      - Flex/ extend digital joints:_____ ☐NAF
      - Flex/ extend/ varus/ valgus of tarsal joints:_____ ☐NAF
      - Palpation of achilles tendon:
        - During flexion of tarsal and stifle joints:_____ ☐NAF
        - During extension of tarsal and stifle joints:_____ ☐NAF
      - Palpation of stifle joint:
        - Patellar luxation: ☐yes, ☐no _____
        - Cranial drawer: ☐yes, ☐no _____
        - Cranial tibial thrust: ☐yes, ☐no _____

    - ○ *Left Pelvic Limb:*
      - Footpads/ interdigital webs:_____ ☐NAF
      - Flex/ extend digital joints:_____ ☐NAF
      - Flex/ extend/ varus/ valgus of tarsal joints:_____ ☐NAF
      - Palpation of achilles tendon:
        - During flexion of tarsal and stifle joints:_____ ☐NAF
        - During extension of tarsal and stifle joints:_____ ☐NAF
      - Palpation of stifle joint:
        - Patellar luxation: ☐yes, ☐no _____
        - Cranial drawer: ☐yes, ☐no _____
        - Cranial tibial thrust: ☐yes, ☐no _____

    - ○ *Right Hip & Pelvis:*
      - Flexion/ extension of hip joint:_____ ☐NAF
      - ± Abduction of hip joint:_____ ☐NAF
      - Ortolani sign: ☐yes, ☐no _____

    - ○ *Left Hip & Pelvis:*
      - Flexion/ extension of hip joint:_____ ☐NAF
      - ± Abduction of hip joint:_____ ☐NAF
      - Ortolani sign: ☐yes, ☐no _____

Orthopedic Examination:

- **Patient**:_____

- **Date**:_____

- General Appearance:
  - ○ Disposition:_____
  - ○ Weight status:_____
  - ○ Limb alignment:_____
  - ○ Positive (failed) sit test: ☐yes, ☐no _____
  - ○ Overt:
    - ▪ Lameness: _____ ☐NAF
    - ▪ Asym. joint swellings:_____ ☐NAF
    - ▪ Asym. soft tis. Swellings:_____ ☐NAF
    - ▪ Muscle atrophy:_____ ☐NAF

- Gait evaluation:
  [*Abnormality examples*: shortened stride, dragging of the toe-nails, toeing-in or toeing-out, limb circumduction, long-strided gait, meniscal click, head bob, *stumbling, *ataxia, *tetraparesis, or *paraparesis (*findings that suggest neuro)]
  - ○ Abnormalities at walk: ☐None, Other:_____
  - ○ Abnormalities at trot: ☐None, Other:_____

- Standing Palpation:
  [*Abnormality examples*: jt. effusion or thickening (medial buttress), heat, malalignment of bony landmarks, crepitus, atrophy]
  - ○ *Thoracic Limb*:
    - ▪ Acromion:_____ ☐NAF
    - ▪ Spine of scapula:_____ ☐NAF
    - ▪ G. tubercle of hum.:_____ ☐NAF
    - ▪ Hum. epicondyles:_____ ☐NAF
    - ▪ Olecranon:_____ ☐NAF
    - ▪ Acc. carpal bn.:_____ ☐NAF
    - ▪ Conscious proprioception:_____ ☐NAF

  - ○ *Pelvic Limb*:
    - ▪ Normal triangular orientation of ilial wing, tuber ischii, and greater trochanter:
      ☐yes, ☐no [Linear orientation of landmarks indicates craniodorsal hip luxation.]
    - ▪ Iliac crest:_____ ☐NAF
    - ▪ Ischiatic tuberosity:_____ ☐NAF
    - ▪ G. trochanter of fem.:_____ ☐NAF
    - ▪ Quadriceps m.:_____ ☐NAF
    - ▪ Patella/ patellar ten.:_____ ☐NAF
      - • Able to define cranial 2/3 of patellar tendon: ☐yes, ☐no _____
      - • Patellar luxation: ☐yes, ☐no _____
        ☐1(In-Out-In), ☐2(In-Out-Out), ☐3(Out-In-Out), ☐4(Out-Out-Out)
    - ▪ Tibial tuberosity:_____ ☐NAF
    - ▪ Hamstring mm.:_____ ☐NAF
    - ▪ Femoral condyles:_____ ☐NAF
    - ▪ Distal tibia:_____ ☐NAF
    - ▪ Achilles tendon:_____ ☐NAF
    - ▪ Tuber calcaneous:_____ ☐NAF
    - ▪ Tarsal joint:_____ ☐NAF
    - ▪ Conscious proprioception:_____ ☐NAF

  - ○ *Vertebral Column*:
    - ▪ Spinal hyperesthesia: ☐yes, ☐no _____
    - ▪ Tail pain: ☐yes, ☐no _____
    - ▪ Sacroiliac jt. pain: ☐yes, ☐no _____

- <u>Recumbent Palpation</u>:
  - [*Abnormality examples*: CREPI – crepitus, decreased range-of-motion, effusion, pain, instability]
  - ○ *Right Thoracic Limb*:
    - ▪ Footpads/ interdigital webs:_____ ☐NAF
    - ▪ Flex/ extend digital joints:_____ ☐NAF
    - ▪ Flex/ extend/ varus/ valgus of carpal joints:_____ ☐NAF
    - ▪ Flex/ extend elbow joint:_____ ☐NAF
    - ▪ Int./ ext. rotation of elbow w/ med. digital pres.:_____ ☐NAF
    - ▪ Flex/ extend shoulder joint:_____ ☐NAF

  - ○ *Left Thoracic Limb*:
    - ▪ Footpads/ interdigital webs:_____ ☐NAF
    - ▪ Flex/ extend digital joints:_____ ☐NAF
    - ▪ Flex/ extend/ varus/ valgus of carpal joints:_____ ☐NAF
    - ▪ Flex/ extend elbow joint:_____ ☐NAF
    - ▪ Int./ ext. rotation of elbow w/ med. digital pres.:_____ ☐NAF
    - ▪ Flex/ extend shoulder joint:_____ ☐NAF

  - ○ *Right Pelvic Limb*:
    - ▪ Footpads/ interdigital webs:_____ ☐NAF
    - ▪ Flex/ extend digital joints:_____ ☐NAF
    - ▪ Flex/ extend/ varus/ valgus of tarsal joints:_____ ☐NAF
    - ▪ Palpation of achilles tendon:
      - • During flexion of tarsal and stifle joints:_____ ☐NAF
      - • During extension of tarsal and stifle joints:_____ ☐NAF
    - ▪ Palpation of stifle joint:
      - • Patellar luxation: ☐yes, ☐no _____
      - • Cranial drawer: ☐yes, ☐no _____
      - • Cranial tibial thrust: ☐yes, ☐no _____

  - ○ *Left Pelvic Limb*:
    - ▪ Footpads/ interdigital webs:_____ ☐NAF
    - ▪ Flex/ extend digital joints:_____ ☐NAF
    - ▪ Flex/ extend/ varus/ valgus of tarsal joints:_____ ☐NAF
    - ▪ Palpation of achilles tendon:
      - • During flexion of tarsal and stifle joints:_____ ☐NAF
      - • During extension of tarsal and stifle joints:_____ ☐NAF
    - ▪ Palpation of stifle joint:
      - • Patellar luxation: ☐yes, ☐no _____
      - • Cranial drawer: ☐yes, ☐no _____
      - • Cranial tibial thrust: ☐yes, ☐no _____

  - ○ *Right Hip & Pelvis*:
    - ▪ Flexion/ extension of hip joint:_____ ☐NAF
    - ▪ ± Abduction of hip joint:_____ ☐NAF
    - ▪ Ortolani sign: ☐yes, ☐no _____

  - ○ *Left Hip & Pelvis*:
    - ▪ Flexion/ extension of hip joint:_____ ☐NAF
    - ▪ ± Abduction of hip joint:_____ ☐NAF
    - ▪ Ortolani sign: ☐yes, ☐no _____

Orthopedic Examination:

- **Patient**:_____

- **Date**:_____

- General Appearance:
  - ○ Disposition:_____
  - ○ Weight status:_____
  - ○ Limb alignment:_____
  - ○ Positive (failed) sit test: ☐yes, ☐no _____
  - ○ Overt:
    - ▪ Lameness: _____ ☐NAF
    - ▪ Asym. joint swellings:_____ ☐NAF
    - ▪ Asym. soft tis. Swellings:_____ ☐NAF
    - ▪ Muscle atrophy:_____ ☐NAF

- Gait evaluation:
  [*Abnormality examples*: shortened stride, dragging of the toe-nails, toeing-in or toeing-out, limb circumduction, long-strided gait, meniscal click, head bob, *stumbling, *ataxia, *tetraparesis, or *paraparesis (*findings that suggest neuro)]
  - ○ Abnormalities at walk: ☐None, Other:_____
  - ○ Abnormalities at trot: ☐None, Other:_____

- Standing Palpation:
  [*Abnormality examples*: jt. effusion or thickening (medial buttress), heat, malalignment of bony landmarks, crepitus, atrophy]
  - ○ *Thoracic Limb*:
    - ▪ Acromion:_____ ☐NAF
    - ▪ Spine of scapula:_____ ☐NAF
    - ▪ G. tubercle of hum.:_____ ☐NAF
    - ▪ Hum. epicondyles:_____ ☐NAF
    - ▪ Olecranon:_____ ☐NAF
    - ▪ Acc. carpal bn.:_____ ☐NAF
    - ▪ Conscious proprioception:_____ ☐NAF

  - ○ *Pelvic Limb*:
    - ▪ Normal triangular orientation of ilial wing, tuber ischii, and greater trochanter:
      ☐yes, ☐no [Linear orientation of landmarks indicates craniodorsal hip luxation.]
    - ▪ Iliac crest:_____ ☐NAF
    - ▪ Ischiatic tuberosity:_____ ☐NAF
    - ▪ G. trochanter of fem.:_____ ☐NAF
    - ▪ Quadriceps m.:_____ ☐NAF
    - ▪ Patella/ patellar ten.:_____ ☐NAF
      - • Able to define cranial 2/3 of patellar tendon: ☐yes, ☐no _____
      - • Patellar luxation: ☐yes, ☐no _____
        ☐1(In-Out-In), ☐2(In-Out-Out), ☐3(Out-In-Out), ☐4(Out-Out-Out)
    - ▪ Tibial tuberosity:_____ ☐NAF
    - ▪ Hamstring mm.:_____ ☐NAF
    - ▪ Femoral condyles:_____ ☐NAF
    - ▪ Distal tibia:_____ ☐NAF
    - ▪ Achilles tendon:_____ ☐NAF
    - ▪ Tuber calcaneous:_____ ☐NAF
    - ▪ Tarsal joint:_____ ☐NAF
    - ▪ Conscious proprioception:_____ ☐NAF

  - ○ *Vertebral Column*:
    - ▪ Spinal hyperesthesia: ☐yes, ☐no _____
    - ▪ Tail pain: ☐yes, ☐no _____
    - ▪ Sacroiliac jt. pain: ☐yes, ☐no _____

- <u>Recumbent Palpation:</u>
  [Abnormality examples: CREPI – crepitus, decreased range-of-motion, effusion, pain, instability]
  - *Right Thoracic Limb:*
    - Footpads/ interdigital webs:_____ ☐NAF
    - Flex/ extend digital joints:_____ ☐NAF
    - Flex/ extend/ varus/ valgus of carpal joints:_____ ☐NAF
    - Flex/ extend elbow joint:_____ ☐NAF
    - Int./ ext. rotation of elbow w/ med. digital pres.:_____ ☐NAF
    - Flex/ extend shoulder joint:_____ ☐NAF

  - *Left Thoracic Limb:*
    - Footpads/ interdigital webs:_____ ☐NAF
    - Flex/ extend digital joints:_____ ☐NAF
    - Flex/ extend/ varus/ valgus of carpal joints:_____ ☐NAF
    - Flex/ extend elbow joint:_____ ☐NAF
    - Int./ ext. rotation of elbow w/ med. digital pres.:_____ ☐NAF
    - Flex/ extend shoulder joint:_____ ☐NAF

  - *Right Pelvic Limb:*
    - Footpads/ interdigital webs:_____ ☐NAF
    - Flex/ extend digital joints:_____ ☐NAF
    - Flex/ extend/ varus/ valgus of tarsal joints:_____ ☐NAF
    - Palpation of achilles tendon:
      - During flexion of tarsal and stifle joints:_____ ☐NAF
      - During extension of tarsal and stifle joints:_____ ☐NAF
    - Palpation of stifle joint:
      - Patellar luxation: ☐yes, ☐no _____
      - Cranial drawer: ☐yes, ☐no _____
      - Cranial tibial thrust: ☐yes, ☐no _____

  - *Left Pelvic Limb:*
    - Footpads/ interdigital webs:_____ ☐NAF
    - Flex/ extend digital joints:_____ ☐NAF
    - Flex/ extend/ varus/ valgus of tarsal joints:_____ ☐NAF
    - Palpation of achilles tendon:
      - During flexion of tarsal and stifle joints:_____ ☐NAF
      - During extension of tarsal and stifle joints:_____ ☐NAF
    - Palpation of stifle joint:
      - Patellar luxation: ☐yes, ☐no _____
      - Cranial drawer: ☐yes, ☐no _____
      - Cranial tibial thrust: ☐yes, ☐no _____

  - *Right Hip & Pelvis:*
    - Flexion/ extension of hip joint:_____ ☐NAF
    - ± Abduction of hip joint:_____ ☐NAF
    - Ortolani sign: ☐yes, ☐no _____

  - *Left Hip & Pelvis:*
    - Flexion/ extension of hip joint:_____ ☐NAF
    - ± Abduction of hip joint:_____ ☐NAF
    - Ortolani sign: ☐yes, ☐no _____

Neurological Examination

- **Patient**:_____

- **Date**:_____

- **Neurological History**:
  - *Onset Date*:_____
  - *Duration*:_____
  - *Progression*: (*peracute / acute / chronic / progressive / static*)_____

- **Previous Treatments**:

Drug	Amount	Dose (mg/kg)	Route	Frequency	Duration

- **Observation**:

  - ***Mental Status***:

Alert	Obtunded	Stupor	Coma
(conscious; capable of responding to sensory stimuli)	(↓ interaction with environment; slow response to verbal stimuli)	(unresponsive unless aroused by noxious stimuli)	(complete unresponsiveness to any stimuli)

  - ***Posture***:

Normal	Head Tilt (L / R)	Tremor	Falling	Circling (Tight / Wide) (L / R)

Schiff-Sherrington (rigid extension of forelimbs without forelimb paresis or ataxia; severe, acute T3-L3 myelopathy)	Opisthotonus (backward arching of head, neck, and spine)	Decerebrate (opisthotonus + rigid extension of all limbs + stupor or coma; severe brain stem lesion)	Decerebellate (opisthotonus + rigid extension of fore-limbs + hip flexion + normal mentation; cerebellar lesion)

  - ***Gait***: *Affected Limb(s)*:

Ambulatory (able to stand and walk 10 steps unaided)	Non-ambulatory (unable to stand and walk 10 steps unaided)

Normal	Paraparesis (bilateral weakness of forelimb/ hindlimb)	Paraplegia (bilateral paralysis of forelimb/ hindlimb)	Tetraparesis (weak in all limbs)	Tetraplegia (paralysis of all limbs)

Monoparesis (weak in 1 limb)	Monoplegia (paralysis of 1 limb)	Hemiparesis (weak in fore- and hindlimb of 1 side)	Hemiplegia (paralysis of fore- and hindlimb of 1 side)

Proprioceptive Ataxia (incoordination due to absence of awareness of joint position; commonly seen with paresis/ paralysis; most common type of ataxia)	Cerebellar Ataxia (dysmetria of all limbs; dysmetria is a lack of coordination of movement typified by the undershoot or overshoot of intended position)	Vestib. Ataxia (asymmetric; typified by leaning/ falling/ rolling to 1 side)

  - ***Motor***: Yes (presence of voluntary movement)   No (absence of voluntary movement)

  - ***Urination***: Yes (presence of voluntary urination)   No (absence of voluntary urination)

L	Knuckling	R
	Front	
	Rear	

L	Hopping	R
	Front	
	Rear	

L	Ext. Post. Thrust	R
	Rear	

L	Wheelbarrowing	R
	Visual	
	Non-visual	

(0=absent, 1=hypo, 2=normal, 3=hyper, 4=clonus)

L	Nerve Function	R
	Biceps (C6-C8)	
	Triceps (C7-T1)	
	Extensor Carpi (C7-T1)	
	Withdrawal Forelimb (C6-T2)	
	Patellar (L4-L6)	
	Cranial Tibial (L6-L7)	
	Gastrocnemius (L6-S1)	
	Withdrawal Hindlimb (L5-S1)	
	Perineal (S1-S2)	
	Panniculus	
	Cross Extensor	
	Tail Tone	
	Anal Tone	

Neuroanatomical Localization	
	Generalized neuromuscular
	Spinal cord (C1-C5)
	Spinal cord (C6-T2)
	Spinal cord (T3-L3)
	Spinal cord (L4-Cd5)
	Caudal brainstem (medulla, pons, midbrain)
	Cerebellum
	Fore brain (thalamus and cerebrum)
	Multifocal/ diffuse

(0=absent, 1=hypo, 2=normal)

L	Nerve Function	R
	Vision & Menace (2)	
	Pupil Size (2, 3)	
	Direct PLR (2, 3)	
	Indirect PLR (2, 3)	
	Palpebral (5, 7)	
	Strabismus (8)	
	Physiologic Nystagmus (8)	
	Spontaneous Nystagmus (8)	
	Mastication (5)	
	Facial Sensation (5)	
	Pinnae Sensation (7)	
	Tongue Tone (12)	
	Facial Muscle Symmetry (7)	
	Swallowing (9, 10)	

Hyperesthesia Localization:_____

L	Superficial Pain (skin) (only if no motor)	R
	Fore	
	Hind	

L	Deep Pain (bone) (only if no superf. pain)	R
	Fore	
	Hind	

Muscle Atrophy:_____

L	Muscle Tone (1=hypo, 2=normal, 3=hyper)	R

L	Root Signature (holding up painful limb)	R

Modified Glasgow Coma Scale score:_____

(see page 190 for scoring)

Neurological Examination

- **Patient**:_____

- **Date**:_____

- **Neurological History**:
  - *Onset Date*:_____
  - *Duration*:_____
  - *Progression*: (*peracute / acute / chronic / progressive / static*)_____

- **Previous Treatments**:

Drug	Amount	Dose (mg/kg)	Route	Frequency	Duration

- **Observation**:

  - ***Mental Status***:

Alert (conscious; capable of responding to sensory stimuli)	Obtunded (↓ interaction with environment; slow response to verbal stimuli)	Stupor (unresponsive unless aroused by noxious stimuli)	Coma (complete unresponsiveness to any stimuli)

  - ***Posture***:

Normal	Head Tilt (L / R)	Tremor	Falling	Circling (Tight / Wide) (L / R)
Schiff-Sherrington (rigid extension of forelimbs without forelimb paresis or ataxia; severe, acute T3-L3 myelopathy)	Opisthotonus (backward arching of head, neck, and spine)	Decerebrate (opisthotonus + rigid extension of all limbs + stupor or coma; severe brain stem lesion)	Decerebellate (opisthotonus + rigid extension of fore-limbs + hip flexion + normal mentation; cerebellar lesion)	

  - ***Gait***:   *Affected Limb(s)*:

Ambulatory (able to stand and walk 10 steps unaided)	Non-ambulatory (unable to stand and walk 10 steps unaided)

Normal	Paraparesis (bilateral weakness of forelimb/ hindlimb)	Paraplegia (bilateral paralysis of forelimb/ hindlimb)	Tetraparesis (weak in all limbs)	Tetraplegia (paralysis of all limbs)
Monoparesis (weak in 1 limb)	Monoplegia (paralysis of 1 limb)	Hemiparesis (weak in fore- and hindlimb of 1 side)	Hemiplegia (paralysis of fore- and hindlimb of 1 side)	

Proprioceptive Ataxia (incoordination due to absence of awareness of joint position; commonly seen with paresis/ paralysis; most common type of ataxia)	Cerebellar Ataxia (dysmetria of all limbs; dysmetria is a lack of coordination of movement typified by the undershoot or overshoot of intended position)	Vestib. Ataxia (asymmetric; typified by leaning/ falling/ rolling to 1 side)

  - ***Motor***:   Yes (presence of voluntary movement)   No (absence of voluntary movement)

  - ***Urination***:   Yes (presence of voluntary urination)   No (absence of voluntary urination)

(0=absent, 1=hypo, 2=normal)

L	Knuckling	R
	Front	
	Rear	

L	Hopping	R
	Front	
	Rear	

L	Ext. Post. Thrust	R
	Rear	

L	Wheelbarrowing	R
	Visual	
	Non-visual	

(0=absent, 1=hypo, 2=normal)

L	Nerve Function	R
	Vision & Menace (2)	
	Pupil Size (2, 3)	
	Direct PLR (2, 3)	
	Indirect PLR (2, 3)	
	Palpebral (5, 7)	
	Strabismus (8)	
	Physiologic Nystagmus (8)	
	Spontaneous Nystagmus (8)	
	Mastication (5)	
	Facial Sensation (5)	
	Pinnae Sensation (7)	
	Tongue Tone (12)	
	Facial Muscle Symmetry (7)	
	Swallowing (9, 10)	

(0=absent, 1=hypo, 2=normal, 3=hyper, 4=clonus)

L	Nerve Function	R
	Biceps (C6-C8)	
	Triceps (C7-T1)	
	Extensor Carpi (C7-T1)	
	Withdrawal Forelimb (C6-T2)	
	Patellar (L4-L6)	
	Cranial Tibial (L6-L7)	
	Gastrocnemius (L6-S1)	
	Withdrawal Hindlimb (L5-S1)	
	Perineal (S1-S2)	
	Panniculus	
	Cross Extensor	
	Tail Tone	
	Anal Tone	

Neuroanatomical Localization
Generalized neuromuscular
Spinal cord (C1-C5)
Spinal cord (C6-T2)
Spinal cord (T3-L3)
Spinal cord (L4-Cd5)
Caudal brainstem (medulla, pons, midbrain)
Cerebellum
Fore brain (thalamus and cerebrum)
Multifocal/ diffuse

Hyperesthesia Localization:_____

L	Superficial Pain (skin) (only if no motor)	R
	Fore	
	Hind	

L	Deep Pain (bone) (only if no superf. pain)	R
	Fore	
	Hind	

Muscle Atrophy:_____

L	Muscle Tone (1=hypo, 2=normal, 3=hyper)	R

L	Root Signature (holding up painful limb)	R

Modified Glasgow Coma Scale score:_____

(see page 190 for scoring)

Neurological Examination

- **Patient**:_____

- **Date**:_____

- **Neurological History**:
  - ○ *Onset Date*:_____
  - ○ *Duration*:_____
  - ○ *Progression*: (*peracute / acute / chronic / progressive / static*)_____

- **Previous Treatments**:

Drug	Amount	Dose (mg/kg)	Route	Frequency	Duration

- **Observation**:

  - ○ **Mental Status**:

Alert	Obtunded	Stupor	Coma
(conscious; capable of responding to sensory stimuli)	(↓ interaction with environment; slow response to verbal stimuli)	(unresponsive unless aroused by noxious stimuli)	(complete unresponsiveness to any stimuli)

  - ○ **Posture**:

Normal	Head Tilt (L / R)	Tremor	Falling	Circling (Tight / Wide) (L / R)

Schiff-Sherrington	Opisthotonus	Decerebrate	Decerebellate
(rigid extension of forelimbs without forelimb paresis or ataxia; severe, acute T3-L3 myelopathy)	(backward arching of head, neck, and spine)	(opisthotonus + rigid extension of all limbs + stupor or coma; severe brain stem lesion)	(opisthotonus + rigid extension of fore-limbs + hip flexion + normal mentation; cerebellar lesion)

  - ○ **Gait**: *Affected Limb(s)*:

Ambulatory	Non-ambulatory
(able to stand and walk 10 steps unaided)	(unable to stand and walk 10 steps unaided)

Normal	Paraparesis	Paraplegia	Tetraparesis	Tetraplegia
	(bilateral weakness of forelimb/ hindlimb)	(bilateral paralysis of forelimb/ hindlimb)	(weak in all limbs)	(paralysis of all limbs)

Monoparesis	Monoplegia	Hemiparesis	Hemiplegia
(weak in 1 limb)	(paralysis of 1 limb)	(weak in fore- and hindlimb of 1 side)	(paralysis of fore- and hindlimb of 1 side)

Proprioceptive Ataxia	Cerebellar Ataxia	Vestib. Ataxia
(incoordination due to absence of awareness of joint position; commonly seen with paresis/ paralysis; most common type of ataxia)	(dysmetria of all limbs; dysmetria is a lack of coordination of movement typified by the undershoot or overshoot of intended position)	(asymmetric; typified by leaning/ falling/ rolling to 1 side)

  - ○ **Motor**:

Yes (presence of voluntary movement)	No (absence of voluntary movement)

  - ○ **Urination**:

Yes (presence of voluntary urination)	No (absence of voluntary urination)

(0=absent, 1=hypo, 2=normal)

L	Knuckling	R
	Front	
	Rear	

L	Hopping	R
	Front	
	Rear	

L	Ext. Post. Thrust	R
	Rear	

L	Wheelbarrowing	R
	Visual	
	Non-visual	

(0=absent, 1=hypo, 2=normal, 3=hyper, 4=clonus)

L	Nerve Function	R
	Biceps (C6-C8)	
	Triceps (C7-T1)	
	Extensor Carpi (C7-T1)	
	Withdrawal Forelimb (C6-T2)	
	Patellar (L4-L6)	
	Cranial Tibial (L6-L7)	
	Gastrocnemius (L6-S1)	
	Withdrawal Hindlimb (L5-S1)	
	Perineal (S1-S2)	
	Panniculus	
	Cross Extensor	
	Tail Tone	
	Anal Tone	

Neuroanatomical Localization
Generalized neuromuscular
Spinal cord (C1-C5)
Spinal cord (C6-T2)
Spinal cord (T3-L3)
Spinal cord (L4-Cd5)
Caudal brainstem (medulla, pons, midbrain)
Cerebellum
Fore brain (thalamus and cerebrum)
Multifocal/ diffuse

(0=absent, 1=hypo, 2=normal)

L	Nerve Function	R
	Vision & Menace (2)	
	Pupil Size (2, 3)	
	Direct PLR (2, 3)	
	Indirect PLR (2, 3)	
	Palpebral (5, 7)	
	Strabismus (8)	
	Physiologic Nystagmus (8)	
	Spontaneous Nystagmus (8)	
	Mastication (5)	
	Facial Sensation (5)	
	Pinnae Sensation (7)	
	Tongue Tone (12)	
	Facial Muscle Symmetry (7)	
	Swallowing (9, 10)	

Hyperesthesia Localization:_____

L	Superficial Pain (skin) (only if no motor)	R
	Fore	
	Hind	

L	Deep Pain (bone) (only if no superf. pain)	R
	Fore	
	Hind	

Muscle Atrophy:_____

L	Muscle Tone (1=hypo, 2=normal, 3=hyper)	R

L	Root Signature (holding up painful limb)	R

Modified Glasgow Coma Scale score:_____

(see page 190 for scoring)

Modified Glasgow Coma Scale (MGCS)

		Score
Motor Activity	Normal gait, normal spinal reflexes	6
	Hemiparesis, tetraparesis, or decerebrate rigidity	5
	Recumbent, intermittent extensor rigidity	4
	Recumbent, constant extensor rigidity	3
	Recumbent, constant extensor rigidity with opisthotonus	2
	Recumbent, hypotonia of muscles, depressed or absent spinal reflexes	1
Brainstem Reflexes	Normal pupillary light reflexes and oculocephalic reflexes	6
	Slow pupillary light reflexes and normal to reduced oculocephalic reflexes	5
	Bilateral unresponsive miosis with normal to reduced oculocephalic reflexes	4
	Pinpoint pupils with reduced to absent oculocephalic reflexes	3
	Unilateral, unresponsive mydriasis with reduced to absent oculocephalic reflexes	2
	Bilateral, unresponsive mydriasis with reduced to absent oculocephalic reflexes	1
Level of Consciousness	Occasional periods of alertness and responsive to environment	6
	Depression or delirium, capable of responding but response may be inappropriate	5
	Semicomatose, responsive to visual stimuli	4
	Semicomatose, responsive to auditory stimuli	3
	Semicomatose, responsive only to repeated noxious stimuli	2
	Comatose, unresponsive to repeated noxious stimuli	1

Interpretation of MGCS Score

The *Modified Glasgow Coma Scale (MGCS)* is an objective way to evaluate neurologic function of dogs after traumatic brain injury. The score is a useful way to monitor progression of neurologic deficits, effects of therapeutic measures, and to assess overall prognosis.

Application:
- When possible, the initial neurological examination (including MGCS scale scoring) should occur before any analgesic therapy to allow adequate assessment of the neurologic status.
- Resuscitation is also necessary prior to the neuro exam because shock can affect neurologic status.
- Repeated neurological assessment is recommended every 30–60 minutes after initial presentation and after interventions are made.

Predicting Prognosis	
3-8	Grave
9-14	Guarded
15-18	Good

Other Specific Numbers From Literature	
8	50% mortality within the first 48 hours of traumatic brain injury
≤17	Sensitivity of 82% and a specificity of 87% for predicting non-survival to hospital discharge

• Source: *Textbook of Small Animal Emergency*, First Edition. Edited by Kenneth J. Drobatz, Kate Hopper, Elizabeth Rozanski, and Deborah C. Silverstein. © 2019 John Wiley & Sons, Inc.

Ophthalmology Examination

- **Patient**:_____

- **Date**:_____

- **Ophthalmic History**:
  - ○ *Onset Date*:_____
  - ○ *Duration*:_____
  - ○ *Progression*: (*peracute / acute / chronic / progressive / static*)_____

- **Previous Treatments**:

Drug	Amount	Dose (mg/kg)	Route	Frequency	Duration

OD (Rt.)	Minimum Database	OS (Lt.)
	Menace	
	Dazzle	
	Direct PLR	
	Indirect PLR	
	Tapetal reflection	
	Palpebral reflex	
	± Corneal reflex	
	Oculocephalic reflex	
	Retropulsion	
	Schirmer tear test (>15 mm/min)*	
	Fluorescein stain uptake	
	Seidel test (+=corneal perforation)	
	Tonometry (10–20 mm Hg)§	
	± Photopic maze (in light)	
	± Scotopic maze (in dark)	
	Aqueous flare (0-4)	

	Lesions on Extraocular Exam and Fundoscopy	
Keratitis	Superficial corneal neovascularization	
	Corneal fibrosis	
	Superficial corneal pigmentation	
	Corneal ulceration	
Conjunctivitis	Mucoid to mucopurulent discharge	
	Blepharospasm	
	Epiphora	
	Conjunctival hyperemia	
	Conjunctival lymphoid follicles	
	Chemosis	
Uveitis	Aqueous flare (pathognomonic)	
	Keratic precipitates (pathognomonic)	
	Hypopyon / hyphema / fibrin (pathognomonic)	
	Miosis	
	Retinal lesions (hemorrhage / hyporeflectivity)	
Glaucoma	Episcleral injection	
	Blepharospasm	
	Corneal edema	
	Mydriasis	
	Optic disc cupping (dark, round, vessels appear on 2 planes)	
	Buphthalmos (enlargement of globe)	
	Lens (sub)luxation (common in terrier breeds)	
Lens Opacity	Nuclear sclerosis (bluish-gray haziness of lens nucleus; tapetal reflection and fundus visible through opacity)	
	Cataract (tapetal reflection not visible through opacity); (<20%=incipient; 20-100%=incomplete; 100%=complete)	
Other	Exophthalmos (protrusion + normal size)	
	Proptosis (protrusion + eyelids caught behind globe equator)	

*Tonometry:
- Lowest reading is most accurate.
- Coefficient of variance should be 95% or 5% based on device.
- <10 mmHg = consistent with uveitis or chronic glaucoma.
- ≥25 mmHg = diagnostic for glaucoma (especially if blind).
- ≥50 mmHg = pressures at which blindness occurs.
- *Contraindications*: ocular trauma (ex., ruptured globe), corneal abrasion or ulcer (do not touch lesion with tonometer), inability to apply topical anesthetics (proparacaine); perform before pupil dilation (tropicamide).

§Schirmer Tear Test:
- <15 mm/min + clinical signs = diagnostic for quantitative KCS.
- ≥15 mm/min + clinical signs = diagnostic for qualitative KCS.
- Clinical signs of KCS are those of keratitis and conjunctivitis.
- *Contraindications*: not performed in cats, deep corneal ulcer, descemetocele, corneal perforation; not necessary with epiphora; perform before any drops or sedation.

Ophthalmology Examination

- **Patient**:_____

- **Date**:_____

- **Ophthalmic History**:
  - ○ *Onset Date*:_____
  - ○ *Duration*:_____
  - ○ *Progression*: (*peracute / acute / chronic / progressive / static*)_____

- **Previous Treatments**:

Drug	Amount	Dose (mg/kg)	Route	Frequency	Duration

OD (Rt.)	Minimum Database	OS (Lt.)
	Menace	
	Dazzle	
	Direct PLR	
	Indirect PLR	
	Tapetal reflection	
	Palpebral reflex	
	± Corneal reflex	
	Oculocephalic reflex	
	Retropulsion	
	Schirmer tear test (>15 mm/min)*	
	Fluorescein stain uptake	
	Seidel test (+=corneal perforation)	
	Tonometry (10–20 mm Hg)§	
	± Photopic maze (in light)	
	± Scotopic maze (in dark)	
	Aqueous flare (0-4)	

	Lesions on Extraocular Exam and Fundoscopy	
Keratitis	Superficial corneal neovascularization	
	Corneal fibrosis	
	Superficial corneal pigmentation	
	Corneal ulceration	
Conjunctivitis	Mucoid to mucopurulent discharge	
	Blepharospasm	
	Epiphora	
	Conjunctival hyperemia	
	Conjunctival lymphoid follicles	
	Chemosis	
Uveitis	Aqueous flare (pathognomonic)	
	Keratic precipitates (pathognomonic)	
	Hypopyon / hyphema / fibrin (pathognomonic)	
	Miosis	
	Retinal lesions (hemorrhage / hyporeflectivity)	
Glaucoma	Episcleral injection	
	Blepharospasm	
	Corneal edema	
	Mydriasis	
	Optic disc cupping (dark, round, vessels appear on 2 planes)	
	Buphthalmos (enlargement of globe)	
	Lens (sub)luxation (common in terrier breeds)	
Lens Opacity	Nuclear sclerosis (bluish-gray haziness of lens nucleus; tapetal reflection and fundus visible through opacity)	
	Cataract (tapetal reflection not visible through opacity); (<20%=incipient; 20-100%=incomplete; 100%=complete)	
Other	Exophthalmos (protrusion + normal size)	
	Proptosis (protrusion + eyelids caught behind globe equator)	

*Tonometry:
- Lowest reading is most accurate.
- Coefficient of variance should be 95% or 5% based on device.
- <10 mmHg = consistent with uveitis or chronic glaucoma.
- ≥25 mmHg = diagnostic for glaucoma (especially if blind).
- ≥50 mmHg = pressures at which blindness occurs.
- *Contraindications*: ocular trauma (ex., ruptured globe), corneal abrasion or ulcer (do not touch lesion with tonometer), inability to apply topical anesthetics (proparacaine); perform before pupil dilation (tropicamide).

§Schirmer Tear Test:
- <15 mm/min + clinical signs = diagnostic for quantitative KCS.
- ≥15 mm/min + clinical signs = diagnostic for qualitative KCS.
- Clinical signs of KCS are those of keratitis and conjunctivitis.
- *Contraindications*: not performed in cats, deep corneal ulcer, descemetocele, corneal perforation; not necessary with epiphora; perform before any drops or sedation.

Ophthalmology Examination

- **Patient**:_____

- **Date**:_____

- **Ophthalmic History**:
  - ○ *Onset Date*:_____
  - ○ *Duration*:_____
  - ○ *Progression*: (*peracute / acute / chronic / progressive / static*)_____

- **Previous Treatments**:

Drug	Amount	Dose (mg/kg)	Route	Frequency	Duration

OD (Rt.)	Minimum Database	OS (Lt.)
	Menace	
	Dazzle	
	Direct PLR	
	Indirect PLR	
	Tapetal reflection	
	Palpebral reflex	
	± Corneal reflex	
	Oculocephalic reflex	
	Retropulsion	
	Schirmer tear test (>15 mm/min)*	
	Fluorescein stain uptake	
	Seidel test (+=corneal perforation)	
	Tonometry (10–20 mm Hg)§	
	± Photopic maze (in light)	
	± Scotopic maze (in dark)	
	Aqueous flare (0-4)	

	Lesions on Extraocular Exam and Fundoscopy	
Keratitis	Superficial corneal neovascularization	
	Corneal fibrosis	
	Superficial corneal pigmentation	
	Corneal ulceration	
Conjunctivitis	Mucoid to mucopurulent discharge	
	Blepharospasm	
	Epiphora	
	Conjunctival hyperemia	
	Conjunctival lymphoid follicles	
	Chemosis	
Uveitis	Aqueous flare (pathognomonic)	
	Keratic precipitates (pathognomonic)	
	Hypopyon / hyphema / fibrin (pathognomonic)	
	Miosis	
	Retinal lesions (hemorrhage / hyporeflectivity)	
Glaucoma	Episcleral injection	
	Blepharospasm	
	Corneal edema	
	Mydriasis	
	Optic disc cupping (dark, round, vessels appear on 2 planes)	
	Buphthalmos (enlargement of globe)	
	Lens (sub)luxation (common in terrier breeds)	
Lens Opacity	Nuclear sclerosis (bluish-gray haziness of lens nucleus; tapetal reflection and fundus visible through opacity)	
	Cataract (tapetal reflection not visible through opacity); (<20%=incipient; 20-100%=incomplete; 100%=complete)	
Other	Exophthalmos (protrusion + normal size)	
	Proptosis (protrusion + eyelids caught behind globe equator)	

*Tonometry:
- Lowest reading is most accurate.
- Coefficient of variance should be 95% or 5% based on device.
- <10 mmHg = consistent with uveitis or chronic glaucoma.
- ≥25 mmHg = diagnostic for glaucoma (especially if blind).
- ≥50 mmHg = pressures at which blindness occurs.
- *Contraindications*: ocular trauma (ex., ruptured globe), corneal abrasion or ulcer (do not touch lesion with tonometer), inability to apply topical anesthetics (proparacaine); perform before pupil dilation (tropicamide).

§Schirmer Tear Test:
- <15 mm/min + clinical signs = diagnostic for quantitative KCS.
- ≥15 mm/min + clinical signs = diagnostic for qualitative KCS.
- Clinical signs of KCS are those of keratitis and conjunctivitis.
- *Contraindications*: not performed in cats, deep corneal ulcer, descemetocele, corneal perforation; not necessary with epiphora; perform before any drops or sedation.

[Intentionally Left Blank]

Specific

Questions

&

References

- ## ACUTE ABDOMEN:

  - Has he/she received any medication, including OTC drugs (ex., aspirin, ibuprofen, etc.)?

  - Is he/she current on vaccinations?

  - Has he/she been exposed to any other animals?

  - Do you have other animals that are ill?

  - What is his/her normal diet?

  - Is it possible that he/she ingested anything unusual (ex., foreign body, toxin, new food)?

  - Is he/she fed bones? If so, what kind and when?

  - Is he/she fed people food? If so, what kind and when?

  - When did he/she last eat?

  - Is he/she urinating normally?

  - Is he/she defecating normally?

  - Is there a possibility of trauma?

  - Does he/she have any history of medical problems?

  - When was she/she last normal?

  - Describe the first sign of abnormality.

  - Describe the progression of abnormal signs.

  - Describe the vomitus:
    - Appearance of contents
    - Volume of contents
    - Frequency of vomiting
  - Aside from the vomiting, is he/she acting normally?

  - Have you noticed any other signs besides vomiting?

Physical Examination:
- Presence of linear foreign body under the tongue?
- Carefully abdominal palpation for:
  - Organomegaly or other palpable masses
  - Gaseous distention
  - Fluid wave
  - Uterine distention
  - Urinary bladder size
  - Localization of pain
- Signs of external trauma?
- Presence and amount of abdominal borborygmus?
  - ↑ Usually seen with acute enteritis, toxicity, and acute intestinal obstruction.
  - ↓ Usually seen with peritonitis, ileus and chronic intestinal obstruction.
- Rectal examination of prostate, lymph nodes, and feces

- ## ANEMIA:

  <u>History</u>:
  - Clinical signs?
    - Lethargy, weakness, exercise intolerance, collapse, inappetence, abnormal color of urine or feces, "coffee ground" appearance of vomitus, pica (suggests chronic anemia)?

  - Medications/ Toxins:
    - that may cause IMHA – recent vaccination, penicillin, sulfa drugs, cephalosporin, other
    - that may affect RBC production – estrogen, phenylbutazone, TMS, chloramphenicol, chemotherapy
    - that may cause oxidative hemolysis – *Allium* species (onion, garlic), acetaminophen (Tylenol), zinc (US pennies minted after 1982, bolts, screws, topical skin protectants), benzocaine, propylene glycol, methylene blue, naphthalene, DL-methionine, phenacetin, phenazopyridine

  - Tick or flea exposure?

  - Past illnesses? – any infection (especially tick-borne disease, erythroparasites, *Dirofilaria*, *Leptospira*, *Clostridium*, endotoxemia), any cancer (especially lymphoma and hemangiosarcoma)

  <u>Physical Examination</u>:
  - Tachycardia, tachypnea, cardiac murmur, gallop heart sound, pallor, jaundice, splenomegaly, pigmenturia, melena, hematochezia, ticks or fleas, retinal hemorrhage, petechia/ ecchymoses, abdominal fluid wave, prostatomegaly, testicular mass?

  <u>Diagnostic/Therapeutic Workup</u>:
  1. Flow-by oxygen
  2. Catheter placement
  3. Pretreatment blood sampling:
     - Red top (Serum), Purple top (EDTA), Blue top (Na Citrate)
     - PCV/TS (± glucose, lactate, BUN, electrolytes, blood gasses)
     - Blood smear with platelet estimate – Polychromasia, anisocytosis, and nRBCs (suggest regenerative anemia), Spherocytes (start treatment for IMHA in dogs), Erythrophagocytosis (start treatment for IMHA), Heinz bodies or Eccentrocytes (start treatment for oxidative hemolysis if history of exposure), Erythroparasites (*Mycoplasma*, *Cytauxzoon*, *Babesia*), Schistocytes (suggests microangiopathic hemolysis secondary to DIC, hemangiosarcoma, *Dirofilaria*, splenic torsion)
  4. Initial stabilization
  5. Diagnostic workup:
     - CBC with reticulocyte count
     - ± Blood typing
     - ± aFAST and tFAST
     - ± Saline agglutination test if suspect hemolysis – start treatment for IMHA if positive
     - ± Direct Coombs test if suspect hemolysis – start treatment for IMHA if positive
     - ± Serum biochemistry – bilirubinemia, uremia of renal or gastric disease, hypophosphatemia (<1.5–2 mg/dL)
     - ± Urinalysis (free catch if spontaneous bleeding) – bilirubinuria, hemoglobinuria, hematuria, anemia of chronic renal disease, UTI
     - ± Urine culture – rule out UTI (especially in IMHA)
     - ± Fecal examination – rule out gastrointestinal parasitism
     - ± Infectious disease testing – FeLV, tick-borne pathogen testing via serology and/or PCR, *Mycoplasma* PCR
     - ± Thoracic and abdominal rads and/or ultrasound – neoplasia, infectious disease, metallic foreign body
     - ± Endocrine testing – hypothyroidism, hypoadrenocorticism
     - ± Gastrointestinal endoscopy – gastrointestinal hemorrhage
     - ± Additional coagulation testing – PT/aPTT, BMBT, D-dimers, viscoelastic testing
     - ± Bone marrow sampling and analysis

  <u>Predispositions</u>:
  - IMHA – cocker spaniel, miniature schnauzer, poodle, English springer spaniel, Old English sheepdog
  - Copper toxicosis – Bedlington terrier, Labrador retriever
  - Babesiosis – greyhound (*B. canis*), pit bull terrier or recent dog bite wound (*B. gibsoni*)
  - Pyruvate kinase deficiency – basenjis, beagle, dachshund, toy Eskimo, West Highland white terrier, cairn terrier
  - Phosphofructokinase deficiency – cocker spaniel, English springer spaniel
  - Hereditary stomatocytosis – standard and miniature schnauzer, Alaskan malamute, Drentsche patrijshound
  - Severe osmotic fragility – Somali, Abyssinian, and Siamese cats

    - Sources: 1, 8

- # BLUNT THORACIC TRAUMA (BTT):

  - Initial Stabilization

  - Diagnostic Workup for BTT Patients:
    - 1st Tier Diagnostics:
      - Triage examination (ABCs)
      - Pulse oximetry
      - Electrocardiogram (ECG)
      - PCV/TS
      - Blood gases
      - Lactate

    - 2nd Tier Diagnostics:
      - Physical examination (*see below*)
      - aFAST, tFAST, vetBLUE
      - Electrolyte quantification
      - Arterial blood pressure

    - 3rd Tier Diagnostics:
      - Complete blood count (CBC)
      - Chemistry panel
      - Coagulation panel (PT/aPTT) ± viscoelastic testing
      - Troponin I (rule in/out myocardial damage)
      - Echocardiogram
      - Fluid analysis (if evidence of effusion)
      - Thoracic radiographs

    - 4th Tier Diagnostics:
      - Computed tomography (CT)
      - Magnetic resonance imaging (MRI)
      - Bronchoscopy
      - Esophagoscopy

  - Physical exam (A CRASH PLAN) – performed as soon as the animal is, or is thought to be, stable:
    - A – Airway: auscultation, oral cavity, pharynx, neck
    - CR – Cardiovascular and Respiratory: auscultation, thorax, respiratory rate monitoring
    - A – Abdomen: gut sounds, bruising, Cullen sign (umbilical ecchymosis), clip hair PRN
    - S – Spine
    - H – Head: eyes, ears, nose, oral cavity (teeth and tongue), cranial nerve exam, modified Glasgow
    - P – Pelvis: perineum, perianal, and rectal examination; external genitalia
    - L – Limbs: skin, muscle, tendon, bone, joint
    - A – Arteries: brachial and femoral pulses; cranial tibial, superficial palmar, and caudal coccygeal
    - N – Nerves: motor and sensory of the limbs and tail

  - Prognosis:
    - Survival to discharge from hospital in dogs with BTT = 88% (n=235).
      - *Negative prognostic indicator*: head trauma, respiratory signs (ex., ARDS, pneumonia, cough, need for mechanical ventilation), hematochezia, lateral recumbency, multi-organ dysfunction.

    - Survival to discharge from hospital in cats with BTT = 90–97%.
      - *Negative prognostic indicator*: flail chest, pleural effusion, diaphragmatic hernia.

  - Conditions associated with BTT:
    - Common: rib fracture, pulmonary contusion, pneumothorax, hemothorax, abnormal ECG
    - Less Common: flail chest, tracheal avulsion, diaphragmatic hernia, pneumomediastinum, ARDS

    - Source: 8, 11

- ## COLLAPSE / SYNCOPE / SEIZURE:

  - Has he/she had single or multiple seizures/collapsing events? Frequency?

  - At what time did the seizure/collapsing event occur?

  - Can you think of anything that may have triggered the seizure/collapsing event?

  - Was he/she exercising or excited before the seizure/collapsing event?

  - Describe how he/she behaved _before_ (1–24 hours prior to) the seizure/collapsing event(s):
    - **Pre-ictal signs**: change in mood or behavior, anxious, restless, hiding, clinging to owner, following owner; may be seen 1–24 hours prior to seizure activity.

  - Describe how he/she behaved _during_ the seizure/collapsing event:
    - Did he/she remain conscious?
      [Note: Animals eyes often remain open when unconscious and this can be misinterpreted as being conscious (their pet was "staring at them").]

    - Did he/she react to being touched or called?

    - Did he/she salivate excessively?

    - Did he/she jaw chomp or teeth chatter?

    - Describe what he/she was doing with his/her limbs during the seizure/collapsing event?
      - Was he/she motionless (sleep-like) with flaccid limb and body tone?
      - Was he/she flailing his/her limbs (as if struggling to get up)?
      - Was he/she repetitively paddling his/her limbs (as if swimming)?

    - About how long did the seizure/collapsing event last (in minutes)?

    - About how long did it take before he/she had completely recovered, physically and mentally?

  - Describe how he/she behaved _after_ (up to 72 hours after) the seizure/collapsing event(s):
    - **Post-ictal signs**: anxious (± wandering, pacing, or running), hyperactive, confused (± ataxic, bumping into things), unresponsive to owner, loss of house training, depressed (can last for days or weeks), lethargic and sleeping a lot, impaired vision/ lack of menace, increased hunger/ thirst.

	Seizure	Syncope
Pre-/ Post-ictal behavior changes	✓	–
Jaw chomping/ teeth chattering	✓	–
Hypersalivation	✓	–
Facial muscle twitching	✓	–
Exhaustion on recovery	✓	–
Opisthotonus	✓	✓
Loss of bladder and/or bowel control	✓	✓
Vocalization	✓	✓
Duration of "collapsing event"	Seconds to minutes	Seconds to minutes
Duration of recovery until 100% normal	Hours-to-days	≤1 Minute
Trigger event	Usually occur at rest or from sleep with no trigger	Often triggered by excitement or onset of exercise
Limbs	• Repetitive paddling/ swimming • Transient forelimb rigidity (also seen in syncope)	• Motionless (sleep-like) with flaccid limb and body tone (more common) • Limb flailing (as if struggling to get up) in partially conscious animals (may mimic seizure) • Transient forelimb rigidity (also seen in epileptic seizures)

- Source: 8, 9

- **DIARRHEA:**

History
Onset – When did the diarrhea start? Does he/she have a history of recurrent bouts of diarrhea?
Exposure – Recent contact with sick animals? Recently boarded? Recent traveling or show attendance?
Dietary Indiscretion – New medications? New foods? Raw or undercooked meat? Tendency to eat inappropriate objects? Missing toys?
Appearance – Describe the appearance of the diarrhea (color and consistency; water *vs.* soft-serve ice cream *vs.* cylindrical)?

	Small Bowel	Large Bowel
Frequency – How many times does it occur in a 24-hour period?	Normal or mild ↑	Severe ↑
Volume – Does the total volume of feces seem greater than normal?	↑ (large volumes of watery diarrhea)	Normal or mild ↑
Urge – Just prior defecating, does he/she show a sense of urgency?	–	Common
Dyschezia – While defecating, does it seem painful or difficult to finish?	–	Common
Tenesmus – While defecating, is there useless or painful straining?	–	Common
Mucous – Any mucous?	–	Common
Hematochezia – Any blood?	–	Occasional
Melena – Has the diarrhea appeared dark and sticky (almost like tar)?	Rare	–
Weight loss – Any recent change in body weight?	Common (especially if chronic)	Uncommon (unless severe disease)
Polyphagia – Any recent change in appetite?	Common	Uncommon
Vomiting – Any recent vomiting?	Occasional	Occasional (10– 20% of cases)

	Acute	Chronic Small Bowel	Chronic Large Bowel
Duration	< 14 days (acute, non-episodic)	≥ 14 days	≥ 14 days

DDX	• Gastrointestinal:
	  ○ Intussusception
	  ○ Food intolerance/ allergy
	  ○ Dietary indescretion/ rapid dietary change
	  ○ Bacterial food poisoning
	  ○ Cytokines (i.e., inflammation, sepsis)
	  ○ Helminths (hook, round, whip, *Strongyloides*, heartworm [especially cats])
	  ○ Bacteria (*Salmonella, Clostridium, E. coli, Campylobacter, Y. enterocolitica*, others)
	  ○ Protozoa (*Giardia, Trichomonas, Cystoisospora, Cryptosporidium*)
	  ○ Virus (CPV, FPV, FeLV, FIV, CDV, Coronavirus, Rotavirus)
	  ○ Rickettsia (Salmon Poisoning)
	  ○ Acute hemorrhagic diarrhea syndrome
	  ○ Stress colitis (dog > cat)
	  ○ Foreign body
	• Systemic:
	  ○ Addison's (Hypoadrenocorticism)
	  ○ Pyometra, Peritonitis, Pancreatitis
	  ○ Drugs (Antibiotics, Chemotherapeutics, Anthelmintics, NSAIDs, Digitalis, others)
	  ○ Toxins (Garbage, Spoiled foods, Chocolate, Chemicals, Heavy metals, Toxic plants)
		• Gastrointestinal:
		  ○ Intussusception
		  ○ Food intolerance/ allergy
		  ○ GI lymphoma (cats)
		  ○ Gastrinoma
		  ○ Inflammatory bowel disease (IBD)
		  ○ Cytokines (i.e., inflammation, sepsis)
		  ○ Helminths (hook, round, whip)
		  ○ Bacteria (SI bacterial overgrowth)
		  ○ Protozoa (*Giardia, Trichomonas, Cystoisospora, Cryptosporidium*)
		  ○ Fungi (*Histoplasma, Pythium*)
		  ○ Intestinal lymphangiectasia
		  ○ Foreign body
		• Systemic:
		  ○ Exocrine pancreatic insufficiency (EPI)
		  ○ Hyperthyroidism (cats)
		  ○ Hypothyroidism (dogs)
		  ○ Liver disease (liver failure, cholestasis)
		  ○ Hyperammonemia (PSS, cirrhosis)
		  ○ Ketones (diabetes, DKA)
		  ○ Uremia (renal failure)
		  ○ Pancreatic carcinoma
		  ○ Head trauma
			• Gastrointestinal:
			  ○ Motility disorders
			  ○ Food intolerance/ allergy
			  ○ Fiber-responsive diarrhea
			  ○ GI Lymphoma (cats)
			  ○ GI Adenocarcinoma (dogs)
			  ○ Inflammatory bowel disease (IBD):
			    · Lymphocytic-plasmacytic colitis
			    · Eosinophilic colitis
			    · Chronic ulcerative colitis
			    · Histiocytic ulcerative colitis (Boxer)
			  ○ Cytokines (i.e., inflammation)
			  ○ Helminths (whip)
			  ○ Bacteria (Clostridial colitis)
			  ○ Protozoa (*Giardia, Trichomonas, Heterobilharzia*)
			  ○ Fungi (*Histoplasma, Pythium*)
			  ○ Virus (FIV/FeLV secondary infection)
			• Systemic:
			  ○ Head trauma

Dx	• *Symptomatic therapy* – reasonable if mild diarrhea, normal demeanor, eating, drinking, no vomiting, and no detectable dehydration.
	• 1st Tier:
	  ○ PCV/TS, BG, BUN, NOVA, Fecal float, Fecal direct smear, SNAP Parvo®
	• 2nd Tier:
	  ○ CBC, Chem, UA, SNAP cPL or fPL®, ACTH-stim (or baseline cortisol), Abd rads, Heartworm Ag and Ab test (cats), GI panel
	• 3rd Tier:
	  ○ Abd US, Endoscopy, Surgical exploratory
	± PT/PTT (if hematochezia/ melena)
		• 1st Tier:
		  ○ Fenbendazole (empirical), Fecal flotation, Fecal direct smear, SNAP *Giardia*®
		  ○ Diet trial with a highly-digestible diet (ex., Hill's i/d, Purina EN, Royal Canin GI)
		• 2nd Tier:
		  ○ CBC, Chemistry, UA, Baseline cortisol, T4 analysis
		  ○ Serum cPL or fPL, GI panel (cTLI, cobalamin, folate), Abdominal rads and US
		  ○ *Cryptosporidium* IFA, *Tritrichomonas* fecal PCR, Fungal EIA for Ag
		• 3rd Tier (therapeutic trials):
		  ○ Parenteral cyanocobalamin (if needed), Diet trial (hydrolyzed Ag or novel protein), Antibiotic trial (tylosin or metronidazole), ± Probiotics, prebiotics, and synbiotics
		• 4th Tier:
		  ○ Abdominal rads and US (if don't already have), Endoscopic biopsy, Surgical biopsy
		  ○ Perform early biopsy if: PLE, severe weight loss with hyporexia, other systemic signs (ex., lymphadenomegaly), melena or hematemesis, or detection of a mass	

- Source: 8, 9, 11

• EMERGENCY:

Waiting Room Triage – Patients that Require Immediate Stabilization	
Respiratory arrest, cardiac arrest	Distended abdomen
Respiratory distress	White, cyanotic, or severely hyperemic mucous membranes
Loss of consciousness, stupor, lateral recumbency	Hyperthermia (>105.8 °F) or history of heat stroke
Status epilepticus, cluster seizures	Hypothermia (<98.1 °F)
Decompensated shock	Dystocia with extruding fetal parts
Bradycardia (cat <120, dog <40–60/min)	Acute poisoning
Tachycardia (cat >240, dog >180)	Stranguria with enlarged and hard bladder (suggestive of urethral obstruction)
Irregular heart rhythm	Snake bites
Arterial hemorrhage	Burns, chemical injury
Perforated or open body cavity	

- Source: 8

Physical Examination Findings at Each Stage of Shock						
	DOG			CAT		
	Compensated Shock	Acute Decompensated Shock	Late Decompensated Shock	Compensated Shock	Acute Decompensated Shock	Late Decompensated Shock
Temp. (°F)	↓ (98–99)	↓↓ (96–98)	↓↓↓ (<96)	↓ (<97)	↓↓ (<95)	↓↓↓ (<90)
HR (bpm)	↑↑ (>180)	↑ (>150)	↓-to-N (<140)	↑↑↑ (>240)	↑↑ (>200)	↑ (>180)
				↓ (160–180)	↓↓ (120–140)	↓↓↓ (<120)
RR (rpm)	↑↑ (>50)	↑ (<50)	N-to-↑-to-Agonal	↑↑↑ (>60)	↑↑ (>60)	↑-to-Agonal
Mentation	QAR	Obtunded	Obtunded-to-Stupor	QAR	Obtunded	Obtunded-to-Stupor
MM color	Pale	Pale	Pale-to-Muddy	Pale	Pale-to-White	Pale-to-White
CRT (sec)	< 1	< 2	≥ 2	< 1	< 2	≥ 2
MAP (mm Hg)	↓-to-N (70–80)	↓ (50–70)	↓↓ (<60)	↓-to-N (80–90)	↓ (50–80)	↓↓ (<50)

- Source: 5

Endpoints of Resuscitation	
Mentation	BAR
Capillary Refill Time	1-2 seconds
Heart Rate	Dog: 70–140; Cat: 140–180 (stressed: 180–220)
Rectal Temperature	100–102 °F
Blood Pressure	SAP >90 mmHg; MAP >60 mmHg
Lactate	< 2 mmol/L

- Source: 4

Fluid Therapy				
Resuscitation	Hydration			
	Fluid Deficit / Dehydration	Maintenance	Ongoing Losses	
• Traditional "shock dose": ◦ **Dog = ¼ of 90 ml/kg** (over 15 min) ◦ **Cat = ¼ of 60 ml/kg** (over 15 min) • Reevaluate based on endpoints of resuscitation.	• **Liters of dehydration = (kg) × (% dehydration)** • Subtract shock bolus volumes from fluid deficit. • Replace over 6–24 hour depending on patient. • Example: ◦ BW = 11 kg ; Estimated Dehydration = 7% ◦ Fluid deficit = (11)(0.07) = 0.77L = 770mL	• Traditional formulas: ◦ **Dog = 40–60 ml/kg/day** ◦ **Cat = 48–72 ml/kg/day** ◦ **Pediatric = 80–120 ml/kg/day** • Accounts for daily fluid losses from feces, skin, breathing, urine.	• Replace measured volumes of: ◦ Vomit ◦ Regurgitation ◦ Diarrhea ◦ Saliva ◦ Draining fluid ◦ Blood loss	

- Subcutaneous fluid dose (outpatient treatment of dehydration with mild clinical signs and normal tissue perfusion parameters): 10–30 mL/kg
- Source: 8

- **EUTHANASIA/ SERIOUS ILLNESS CONVERSATION GUIDE**:

  - UNDERSTANDING:
    - What is your understanding now of where _____ is with his/her illness?

    - What questions do you have about information your family veterinarian has already shared with you?

  - INFORMATION PREFERENCES:
    - How much information about _____'s illness would you like from me?

    - How much additional information do you feel you need to help make decisions?

  - PROGNOSIS

  - GOALS:
    - If _____'s situation worsens, what are your most important goals?

  - FEARS / WORRIES:
    - What are your biggest fears and worries about _____'s health?

  - FUNCTION:
    - What abilities or activities are so critical to _____'s life that you can't imagine him/her living without them?

  - TRADE-OFFS:
    - If _____ becomes sicker, how much are you willing to go through for the possibility of gaining more time together?

  - AID IN DYING:
    - What are your beliefs surrounding euthanasia?

  - KEY PHRASES:
    - Hope for best, prepare for worst

    - My goal is to help you identify the greatest benefit for both _____ and your family.

    - No decision necessary today

    - I wish for [X], too. But I worry that [Y]. So, I wonder if we might be able to talk about a plan B, just in case things don't go the way we want them to.

  - Source: Goldberg, Katherine J. "Goals of Care: Development and Use of the Serious Veterinary Illness Conversation Guide." *Veterinary Clinics of North America: Small Animal Practice*, vol. 49, no. 3, May 2019, pp. 399–415.

- # HEART FAILURE:

Diagnosis of Congestive Heart Failure		
	Dog	**Cat**
Heart Auscultation	• Tachycardia (>150 bpm) • Arrhythmia (but NOT respiratory sinus arrhythmia)* • Murmur • Gallop heart sound	• Tachycardia (>240 bpm) • Arrhythmia* • Murmur • Gallop heart sound
Lung Auscultation	↑ Bronchovesicular sounds	• ↑ Bronchovesicular sounds • Absent/ muffled heart sounds
Pulses	• Weak pulses • Pulse deficit	• Weak pulses • Pulse deficit
Radiographs	• VHS > 10.5 • Pulmonary infiltrate – CHF pattern	• VHS > 8.1 • Pulmonary infiltrate – CHF pattern
Venous Distension	Present at rest	Present at rest
Blood Biomarkers	NT-proBNP > 2500	NT-proBNP ≥ 270
Therapeutic Trials	Clinical and radiographic response to CHF therapy	Clinical and radiographic response to CHF therapy

- * Arrhythmias, including respiratory sinus arrhythmias, can be diagnosed ONLY via ECG. Dogs in heart failure should NOT have a respiratory sinus arrhythmia.
- Diagnosis of CHF made based on these findings; however, there can be inconsistencies. For example, if you have a dog with a murmur, a VHS > 10.5, and a heart rate of 120 bpm (rather than 150), then you need to treat this dog for CHF. If 20 factors support CHF and 2 factors do not support CHF, then go with CHF!
- Source: 10

Heart Failure: Inability of the heart to meet tissue perfusion needs with normal filling pressures.				
	Backward Heart Failure		**Forward Heart Failure**	**Pericardial Effusion**
	Left Ventricular = **cardiogenic pulmonary edema**	**Right Ventricular =** **Ascites (Dog) ±** **Pleural Effusion (Cat)**		
Wet / Cold	Wet	Wet	Cold	–

History	• Acute (< 30 days)
	• Dull/ depressed
	• Anorexia → weight loss
	• Orthopnea
	• Respiratory distress:
	  ∘ Cough
	  ∘ Tachypnea
	  ∘ Dyspnea
	  ∘ ↑ Home resting resp. rate
		• Pot belly/ abdominal distension
		• Diarrhea (due to passive GI congestion)
		• Dyspnea (compression in diaphragm)
		• Tachypnea (compression in diaphragm)
		• Weight loss
		• ↑ Home resting resp. rate
		• Orthopnea
			• Lethargy
			• Dull/ depressed
			• Exercise intolerance
			• Weakness
			• Collapse
			• Syncope
			• Weight loss
				• Cough (secondary to enlarged pericardial sac, resulting in compression of airways)
				• Tachypnea/Dyspnea
				• Exercise intolerance
				• Weakness/ lethargy
				• Abdominal distension
				• Reduced appetite

Physical Exam	• ± Murmur
	• Relative tachycardia
	• Lung sounds:
	  ∘ Normal (possible)
	  ∘ ↑ BV sounds (1°)
	  ∘ Soft crackles (less common)
	  ∘ Soft wheezes (less common)
	
	(Note: ↑ BV sounds are the most common sounds associated with pulmonary edema. Strong crackles are much more likely to be airway disease.)
		• ± Murmur:
		  ∘ Valve disease = murmur
		  ∘ Cardiomyopathy = none
		• ± Relative tachycardia
		• Ascites:
		  ∘ Common in dogs
		  ∘ Rare in cats
		• Jugular distension at rest
		• Positive hepatojugular reflux
		• Pleural effusion (uncommon):
		  ∘ Muffled lung sounds
		  ∘ Muffled heart sounds
			• ± Murmur:
			  ∘ Valve disease = murmur
			  ∘ Cardiomyopathy = none
			• Relative tachycardia
			• Cool extremities
			• Weak pulses
			• Prolonged CRT
			• Cyanosis
			• Low body temperature
				• **Tachycardia**
				• **Hypotension (weak pulses)**
				• **Muffled heart sounds (IMPORTANT)**
				• **Jugular venous distension**
				• Tachypnea
				• Abnormal pulse quality
				  ∘ Pulsus paradoxus – absent palpable pulse during inspiration despite auscultation of a heartbeat
				• Abdominal effusion

Diagnostic Tests	• Thoracic radiographs (best initial diagnostic test if cardiogenic pulmonary edema is suspected)
	• Echocardiogram
	• NT-proBNP
		• Ascites:
		  ∘ Diagnostic abdominocentesis
		  ∘ Echocardiogram
		  ∘ Abdominal ultrasound
		
		• Pleural Effusion:
		  ∘ Thoracic radiographs
		  ∘ Echocardiogram
		  ∘ Diagnostic pleurocentesis
			• Hypotension
			• Prerenal azotemia (elevated BUN and creatinine with adequately concentrated urine)
			• Venous O_2 tension <24 mmHg
			• Increased serum lactate
			• Decreased urine production
				• Echocardiogram (gold standard)
				• Thoracic radiographs
				• ECG:
				  ∘ ± Low-amplitude QRS
				  ∘ ± Electrical alternans
				  ∘ ± VPCs and/or V-tach
				• Pericardiocentesis

- Source: 10

• LIVER ABNORMALITIES / ICTERUS:

Icterus – Direct Liver Pathology vs. Peracute Hemolysis		
	Direct Liver Pathology	**Peracute Hemolysis**
Onset of clinical signs listed below	Several days prior to the onset of icterus	A few hours prior to the onset of icterus
Icterus	✓	✓
Inappetence/ Anorexia	✓	✓
Mental Depression	✓	✓
Lethargy/ Weakness	✓	✓
Vomiting	✓	✓ (sometimes)
Diarrhea	✓	–

• Source: 8

Drugs	**Toxins**
• Drugs associated with ↑ ALT: 　◦ acetaminophen (Tylenol, Dayquil, Nyquil, Excedrin, Robitussin, Theraflu, Vicks) 　◦ amiodarone (Pacerone) 　◦ carprofen (Rimadyl) 　◦ clindamycin (Cleocin) 　◦ doxycycline (Adoxa) 　◦ diazepam (Valium) 　◦ itraconazole (Onmel, Sporanox, Tolsura) 　◦ ketoconazole (Nizoral) 　◦ salicylazosulfapyridine (Azulfidine) 　◦ sulfonamides (sulfamethoxazole/ trimethoprim, sulfisoxazole) • Drugs associated with ↑ ALP: 　◦ anabolic steroids/ androgens (testosterone) 　◦ cephalosporins (cephalexin, cefazolin) 　◦ cyclophosphamide (Cytoxan, Neosar) 　◦ dapsone 　◦ estrogens (estradiol) 　◦ gold salts 　◦ phenothiazines (fluphenazine, chlorpromazine, prochlorperazine) 　◦ progesterone (Prometrium) 　◦ vitamin A (AFirm 1X cream and lotion) • Drugs associated with ↑ ALT and ↑ ALP: 　◦ L-asparaginase 　◦ azathioprine (Imuran, Azasan) 　◦ barbiturates (Seconal, Mebaral) 　◦ erythromycin (EryPed) 　◦ glucocorticoids (only dogs) (cortisone, prednisone, dexamethasone) 　◦ griseofulvin (Grifulvin) 　◦ ibuprofen (Advil, Midol, Motrin) 　◦ mercaptopurine 　◦ methimazole (Tapazole, Northyx) 　◦ methotrexate (Otrexup, Rasuvo, Trexall, Xatmep) 　◦ nitrofurantoin (Furadantin, Macrobid, Macrodantin) 　◦ phenobarbital (Solfoton, Luminal) 　◦ primidone (Mysoline) 　◦ salicylates (Aspirin, Alka-Seltzer) 　◦ tetracycline (Ala-Tet, Brodspec, Panmycin) 　◦ trimethoprim-sulfa drug	• Toxins associated with hemolysis: 　◦ acetaminophen (cats) 　◦ *Allium* spp. (onion, garlic) 　◦ benzocaine 　◦ heavy metals (copper, lead, and zinc [in certain coins after 1982]) 　◦ methylene blue 　◦ mushrooms (specific species) 　◦ propylene glycol 　◦ venom from snakes, brown recluse spiders, and bees • Toxins associated with hepatitis: 　◦ aflatoxin (produced by fungi) 　◦ blue-green algae 　◦ hydrocarbon solvents (benzene, kerosene, xylene) 　◦ melaleuca oil (tea tree oil, which is a type of essential oil) 　◦ mushrooms (*Amanita* spp.) 　◦ sago palm 　◦ xylitol 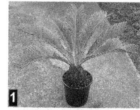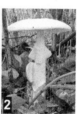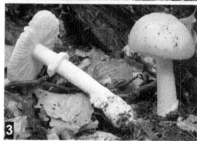 (1) *Cycas revoluta* (sago palm) house plant; (2) *Amanita virosa* (European destroying angel); (3) *Amanita phalloides* (Death Cap)

•　　ALT – alanine aminotransferase; ALP – alkaline phosphatase
•　　Sources: 6, 8

• OBESITY:

- Each animal is classified on a scale of 1 to 5 or 1 to 9 points.

- The 9-point scale establishes ideal weight at 5, with each point above or below representing weight gain or loss of approximately 10-15% (Ettinger, 733).

- Example: Dog with <u>BCS = 8</u> and <u>BW = 30kg</u>

1. $(BCS-5)=(8-5)=3\ BCS\ scores\ overweight$

2. $(Excess\ BCS)(10)=(3)(10)=30\ percent\ overweight$

3. $\dfrac{(Ideal\ BW)}{(BW)}*\dfrac{100-percent\ overweight}{100}=\dfrac{(Ideal\ BW)}{(30\,kg)}*\dfrac{100-30}{100}=21\,kg$

4. $RER(kcal/day)=(30*Ideal\ BW\,[kg])+70=(30*21)+70=700\,kcal/day$

- Source: 9

• TOXIN EXPOSURE:

- ○ The goal of therapy is to "treat the patient, not the poison." Thus, identifying the toxin is not always required for effective therapy.
- ○ The ASPCA Animal Poison Control Center (APCC) is available for consultation 24 hours a day ($65 charge): **(888) 426-4435**

Client Communication / History	Treatment

Telephone Triage Advice:
- Safely remove your pet from the source of toxin exposure.
- Seek immediate veterinary care if the consumed substance is toxic.
- **Do not** use any therapy found on the internet.
- **Do not** induce vomiting unless instructed to do so by an animal poison control center or a veterinarian (see guidelines below).
- Bring the original container or bait station to the veterinarian.
- Estimate the maximum amount of toxin ingested.
- If your pet ingested something caustic (ex., acids or alkalis), then give your pet milk or water to dilute the material, and seek immediate veterinary care.
- Guidelines for recommending at-home induction of emesis in dogs:
  - ○ Canine patients must meet all of the following criteria (only dogs):
    - □ Presence of a valid veterinarian-client-patient relationship.
    - □ No contraindications for induction of emesis.
    - □ No predispositions for aspiration (ex., decreased alertness, laryngeal paralysis, megaesophagus, upper airway disease)
    - □ Transport to hospital will bring the time elapsed since exposure to ≥1–2 hours, making induction of emesis contraindicated.
    - □ Owner is warned that use of oral hydrogen peroxide may result in mucosal irritation, aspiration, or hemorrhagic gastritis; use is recommended only if the dog will have immediate veterinary care.
  - ○ *Dog*: Hydrogen peroxide 3% (only 3% medical grade solution), 2.2 mL/kg, PO (maximum of 45 mL/dog); repeat dose if no vomiting after 15 minutes; do not use in cats, only use in dogs.

Questions to Ask On Presentation After Stabilization:
A) Known Exposure to Toxin:
- Route of exposure (ex., oral, dermal, ocular, inhalation, other)?
- Toxin involved:
  - ○ Product name?
  - ○ Active ingredient(s)?
  - ○ Concentration?
  - ○ Extended-release (ex., Adderall versus Adderall-XR)?
  - ○ Hyphenated brand name (ex., Tylenol versus Tylenol-PM)?
- Maximum amount (ex., total number of pills, total volume of fluid, etc.) of toxin exposure (worst-case scenario)?
- Time of toxin exposure?
- Did you attempt any therapy?
  - ○ Did you attempt to induce vomiting? If yes, what agent was used?
  - ○ Did you offer anything orally (ex., hydrogen peroxide, salt, milk, peanut butter, oil, fat)?
- Clinical signs:
  - ○ Has your pet shown any clinical signs?
  - ○ When was the last time your pet appeared normal?
  - ○ When was the onset of clinical signs?
  - ○ What was the first clinical sign seen? Subsequent clinical signs?

B) Unknown but Suspected Exposure to Toxin:
- Where was your pet prior to the onset of clinical signs?
- Recent (in the last 24 hour) administration of medications, herbal products, essential oils, flea or tick control products to your pet or other animals in the house?
- Recent use of automotive products, solvents, or paints?
- Indoor animal:
  - ○ Human prescription/OTC drugs and herbal products in the house?
  - ○ Veterinary prescription/OTC drugs and herbal products in the house?
  - ○ Recent visitors who may have dropped medications?
  - ○ Household plants? Outdoor plants?
  - ○ Recent use of household cleaner?
  - ○ Recent use of household herbicide, insecticide, or rodenticide?
  - ○ Are other household pets showing any clinical signs?
- Outdoor animal:
  - ○ What are your pet's immediate surroundings?
  - ○ Access to garage, outbuilding, shed, or barn containing potentially toxic substances (ex, fertilizer, herbicide, insecticide, rodenticide, household cleaner, automotive products, paint)?
  - ○ Access to plants, mushrooms, compost piles, or ponds?
- Access to livestock:
  - ○ Access to fly bait?
  - ○ Access to feed bins, medicated feed, or feed with growth promotants?
  - ○ Recent administration of medication or dewormer to livestock?
  - ○ Recent euthanasia and burial of livestock on the property?

Initial Stabilization:
- Assess ABCs and address seizures, hemorrhage, and hyperthermia.
- ± Obtain venous access and draw blood (1 3cc EDTA and 2 serum tubes).

Anti-convulsant Therapy:
- Midazolam (0.2 mg/kg, intranasal) or (0.1 –0.3 mg/kg, IM or slow IV)
- Diazepam (0.5 mg/kg, intranasal) or (0.5–1 mg/kg, slow IV)
- Administer a maximum of 3 anti-convulsant boluses.

GI Decontamination:
A) Induction of Emesis:
- *Dog*: Apomorphine (0.03 mg/kg, IV) or (0.04 mg/kg, IM) or one crushed tablet (6.25 mg) dissolved in water or saline administered into the conjunctival sac. Flush the conjunctival sac with saline post-emesis.
- *Cat*: Xylazine (0.44 mg/kg, IM). Reverse xylazine post-emesis.
- Feeding a small meal (ex., a slice of bread) prior to inducing vomiting can improve emesis.
- Collect vomitus in a glass jar with a tight lid and refrigerate or freeze.
- Contraindications:
  - ■ Symptomatic (ex., CNS depression, respiratory distress, vomiting)
  - ■ ≥1–2 hours since ingestion of most toxins
  - ■ ≥4–6 hours since ingestion of toxins that may take longer to pass (ex., large volume ingestion, chocolate, grapes, gum)
  - ■ Ingestion of corrosive or caustic substances (ex., acids, alkalis)

B) Activated Charcoal (AC):
- Single-dose (and loading-dose) AC therapy:
  - ○ *Drug*: AC with an osmotic cathartic (ex., sorbitol)
  - ○ *Dose*: 1–5 g/kg, PO (the standard dose is 2 g/kg, PO)
  - ○ Single-dose AC therapy may be indicated in animals with a high suspicion of toxin ingestion.
- Multi-dose AC therapy:
  - ○ *Drug*: AC without an osmotic cathartic (due to risk of excessive free water loss into the GI tract and secondary hypernatremia)
  - ○ *Dose*: 1–2 g/kg, PO, q6h for 24 hours (first dose given 6h after an initial loading dose of AC with an osmotic cathartic)
  - ○ *Indications*: Substances that undergo enterohepatic recirculation, extended-release drugs, and drugs with a long half-life
- Contraindications:
  - ○ Patient-related Contraindications:
    - ■ Symptomatic (ex., CNS depression, respiratory distress, vomiting)
    - ■ ≥ 6 hours since ingestion of most toxins
    - ■ Require imminent endoscopy or surgery
    - ■ Gastrointestinal disease (ex., ileus, obstruction, perforation)
    - ■ High risk of aspiration (ex., absent gag reflex, laryngeal paralysis, megaesophagus, upper airway disease)
    - ■ Dehydration or hypovolemia
    - ■ Electrolyte abnormalities (ex., hypernatremia)
    - ■ Hyperosmolar states (ex., renal disease, diabetes mellitus)
  - ○ Toxin-related Contraindications:
    - ■ Corrosive or caustic substances (ex., acids, alkalis)
    - ■ Hydrocarbons or petroleum distillates
    - ■ Salt (ex., homemade play dough, sea water, table salt, paintballs)
    - ■ Substances that do not bind AC (ex., heavy metals, iron salts, fertilizer, nitrates, nitrites, fluoride, iodides, sodium chloride, chlorate, xylitol, ethylene glycol, alcohol, ethanol, methanol)
  - ○ Contraindications for cathartics include diarrhea and dehydration.

Dilution of GI Contents:
- In certain cases, GI contents may be diluted with oral milk or water:
  - ○ *Indications*: Ingestion of corrosive substances or toad secretions, and taste reactions (ex., "foaming kitties" treated with topical flea spray)

Cutaneous Decontamination:
- First, bathe the animal with mild soap shampoo. This should be done at the veterinary hospital if the pet is not alert or is in any kind of distress.
- Administer activated charcoal therapy when indicated (see above).

Ocular Decontamination:
- First, flush the eyes with 2–3 L of physiological saline.
- Treat ocular inflammation and/or ulceration as needed.

• Sources: 1, 3, 7, 8

- **URINARY DISEASE** – **Polyuria/ Abnormal or Inappropriate Urination:**

  - Age at neutering?

  - Age at onset of problem?

  - History of urinary problems? Recent trauma?

  - Frequency of urination? Increased, Normal, or Decreased?
    - If increased:
      - *Recently administered drugs?* (steroids [oral, topical], diuretics, phenobarbital, T4)
      - *Recent change in diet? Increased salt?*
      - *Other signs of illness?*

  - Using hand gestures, what is the *volume* of urine produced with each urination?
    - Large volume (suggests polyuria, pollakiuria)
    - Small volume (suggests stranguria, pollakiuria)

  - Straining? If yes, is any urine being passed?
    - Does he/she ultimately produce a normal volume of urine after making multiple attempts to urinate small volumes of urine? (suggests stranguria)

  - Color of urine? Blood? (clear suggests polyuria)

  - Dribbling? (suggests incontinence; spontaneous voiding when awake suggests urge incontinence)
    - Continuous or intermittent?
    - Intentional or Accidental?
    - Aware of dribbling?
    - Occur at rest? Sleep? Awake? When moving?

  - Change in thirst?

  - If referred:
    - Did the referring vet perform UA or culture?
    - Did the referring vet have you bring in a urine sample or was it collected in-clinic?

- Predispositions:
  - Older cat (suggests hyperthyroidism)
  - Intact female (pyometra)
  - VERY young (primary nephrogenic diabetes insipidus; exclude otherwise)

- KEY TERMS:
  - *Dysuria* – difficult urination (usually associated with pain)
  - *Stranguria* – straining to urinate
  - *Pollakiuria* – increased frequency of urination
  - *Polyuria* – urine production >50 ml/kg/day (polyuric animals are always polydipsic) (cats = ½ volume)
  - *Polydipsia* – water intake >100 ml/kg/day (polydipsic animals are always polyuric) (cats = ½ volume)

- **VESTIBULAR DISEASE**:

  ○ *Minimum Database*: otoscopic exam, oropharyngeal exam (especially cats), CBC, chemistry, urinalysis, and thyroid panel (tT4, fT4, and TSH) ± Schirmer tear test if facial weakness.

Vestibular Disease – Clinical Findings				
	Bilateral Peripheral Vestibular Disease	**Unilateral Peripheral Vestibular Disease**	**Central Vestibular Disease**	**Paradoxical Vestibular Disease**
Mentation	Normal (disoriented if peracute)	Normal (disoriented if peracute)	Normal to comatose	Normal to comatose
Ataxia	• Vestibular ataxia	• Vestibular ataxia	• Vestibular ataxia ± Proprioceptive ataxia ± Cerebellar ataxia	• Vestibular ataxia ± Proprioceptive ataxia ± Cerebellar ataxia
Fall, lean	Toward both sides (symmetrical)	Toward lesion	Toward lesion	Away from lesion
Head tilt	Absent	Toward lesion	Toward lesion	Away from lesion
Circling	Absent	Toward lesion	Toward lesion	Away from lesion
Pathologic nystagmus fast phase	Absent pathologic and physiologic nystagmus	Away from lesion	Away from lesion	Towards lesion
Pathologic nystagmus direction [#]	Absent pathologic and physiologic nystagmus	• Horizontal • Rotary • Vertical (rare but possible)	• Horizontal • Rotary • Vertical ± Positional changes [#]	• Horizontal • Rotary • Vertical ± Positional changes [#]
Other CN deficits	Ipsilateral to falling/ head tilt (ipsilateral to lesion): • CN 7 • Horner's syndrome	Ipsilateral to falling/ head tilt (ipsilateral to lesion): • CN 7 • Horner's syndrome	Ipsilateral to falling/ head tilt (ipsilateral to lesion): • CN 5–12 • Horner's syndrome (rare)	Contralateral to falling/ head tilt (ipsilateral to lesion): • CN 5–12 • Horner's syndrome (rare)
Postural reaction deficits [X]	Absent	Absent	Ipsilateral to falling/ head tilt (ipsilateral to lesion) [X]	Contralateral to falling/ head tilt (ipsilateral to lesion) [X]
Spinal reflexes	Normal	Normal	Normal to increased (UMN)	Normal to increased (UMN)
Palpation	Ear/ facial pain	Ear/ facial pain	± Cervical pain	± Cervical pain

- [#] Positional pathologic (spontaneous) nystagmus may change in character (or may only be present) after a change in head or body position (ex., while pointing the patients snout towards the ceiling, or after placing the patient in dorsal recumbency).
- [X] Postural reactions include conscious proprioception (knuckling) and hopping responses. Postural recreation deficits and paresis helps localize the lesion to the central vestibular system, but absence of these findings does not rule out central vestibular disease.

Vestibular Disease – Differential Diagnoses		
	Peripheral Vestibular	**Central Vestibular**
Degenerative	–	Lysosomal storage disease, Cerebellar cortical abiotrophy
Anomalous	Congenital vestibular disease, Congenital pendular nystagmus	Hydrocephalus, Intracranial intra-arachnoid cyst
Metabolic	Hypothyroidism	Hypothyroidism, Thiamine deficiency (ex., fish diets)
Neoplasia	1° aural neoplasia (squamous cell carcinoma, ceruminous gland adenocarcinoma, sebaceous gland adenocarcinoma), Neurofibrosarcoma, Cholesteatoma	1° intracranial neoplasia (meningioma, glioma, lymphoma, choroid plexus tumors), Metastatic neoplasia (hemangiosarcoma, lymphoma, metastatic carcinoma)
Infectious	Otitis media/interna (*Staphylococcus, Pseudomonas aeruginosa*, beta-hemolytic *Streptococcus, Proteus, E. coli*; **1st most common cause of peripheral vestibular disease in dogs**)	Viral (CDV, FIP, rabies), Bacterial (otogenic, septic meningitis, penetrating trauma), Rickettsial (RMSF, *Ehrlichia*), Protozoal (*Neospora, Toxoplasma*), Fungal (systemic fungi, *Aspergillus*)
Inflammatory	Nasopharyngeal polyp	Meningoencephalitis of unknown etiology (MUE)
Idiopathic	Idiopathic vestibular disease (aka., old dog vestibular disease; **2nd most common cause of peripheral vestibular disease in dogs**), Idiopathic polyneuropathy of CN 7 and 8	–
Toxin	Aminoglycoside, Cisplatin, Loop diuretic, Chlorhexidine, Erythromycin, Chloramphenicol, Minocycline, Five-lined skink	Metronidazole, Lead, Ivermectin
Trauma	Ear flush (iatrogenic), Bulla surgery (iatrogenic), Bulla fracture	Head trauma
Vascular	–	Stroke (ischemic, hemorrhagic), Transient ischemic attack, Feline ischemic encephalopathy

- Source: 8

• VOMITING

History:

- ○ *Onset* – When was the first time you saw him/her vomit?
- ○ *Frequency* – How many times has he/she vomited in the past 24-hours? What is the frequency of vomiting?
- ○ *Volume* – Using hand gestures, what is the average volume produced?
- ○ *Timing*:
  - ▪ Does it occur *variably* without any apparent cause? – suggests vomit
  - ▪ Does it occur only *shortly after* eating/ drinking? – suggests regurge
  - ▪ Does it occur only *while* eating/ drinking? – suggests dysphagia
- ○ *Animal's Expectation*:
  - ▪ Does he/she show discomfort/ anxiety immediately before (as if anticipating vomit)? – suggests vomit
  - ▪ Does it seem completely unexpected? – suggests regurge
  - ▪ Does it occur only while at the food/ water bowl? – suggests dysphagia
- ○ *Activity*:
  - ▪ Does he/she heave out the "vomit" with abdominal contractions (active)? – suggests vomit
  - ▪ Does he/she eject "vomit" suddenly and calmly (passive)? – suggests regurge
  - ▪ Does he/she appear interested in food, but has trouble swallowing? – suggests dysphagia
- ○ Describe the *contents* of the "vomit":
  - ▪ Blood? Coffee grounds appearance?
  - ▪ Does is appear more like:
    - • Digested food (with bile/ yellow, sticky stuff)? – suggests vomit
    - • Undigested food (without bile/ yellow, sticky stuff)? – suggests regurge
    - • Excessive drool or saliva? – suggests dysphagia
- ○ *Dietary Indiscretion*:
  - ▪ New medications? New foods?
  - ▪ Does he/she have a tendency to eat inappropriate objects? Any missing toys?

	Acute, Self-Limiting	**Acute, Potentially Life-Threatening**	**Chronic**
Duration	≤ 7 days	≤ 7 days	>7 days
Character	• Infrequent • History of dietary indescretion • Otherwise normal patient ± Mild abdominal discomfort	• Profuse/ persistent/ increasing frequency ± Hematemesis, fever, severe diarrhea, abdominal pain, not up-to-date on vaccinations	—
DDX	• Gastrointestinal: ○ Intussusception ○ Motion sickness ○ Dietary indescretion (1° dogs) ○ Overeating ○ Parasites (hook, round, whip) ○ Virus (canine coronavirus) ○ Foreign body (irritation; not obstruction) • Systemic: ○ Drugs (Amoxicillin-clavulanate, Chemotherapeutics, Chloramphenicol, Digitalis, Erythromycin, Opioids, Tetracycline, Theophylline, Xylazine)	• Gastrointestinal: ○ Intussusception ○ Dietary indescretion (1° dogs) ○ Parasites (hook, round, whip) ○ Virus (parvo, distemper, panleuk, FIP) ○ Bacteria (*Salmonella*, *Campylobacter*, *Leptospira*, salmon poisoning) ○ Acute hemorrhagic diarrhea syndrome ○ Foreign body (obstruction) ○ Torsion • Systemic: ○ Addison's (hypoadrenocorticism) ○ Hyperammonemia (PSS, cirrhosis) ○ Uremia (renal disease) ○ Ketonemia (DKA) ○ Septicemia/ Peritonitis/ Pyometra ○ Meningitis/ Encephalitis ○ IMHA/ ITP/ IMPA ○ Acute pancreatitis ○ Drugs – *same as left* ○ Toxins (ethylene glycol, mushrooms, organophosphates, pesticides, other)	• Gastrointestinal: ○ Intussusception ○ Partial obstruction ○ Gastrointestinal ulceration ○ Chronic Enteritis (ex., diet responsive) ○ Cancer (lymphoma, carcinoma) ○ Inflammatory bowel disease (IBD) ○ Parasites (*Physaloptera*, *Ollulanus*) ○ Fungi (pythiosis) ○ Chronic pyloric hypertrophy • Systemic: ○ Hyperthyroidism (cats) ○ Hyperammonemia (PSS, cirrhosis) ○ Uremia (chronic renal disease) ○ Hypercalcemia ○ Paraneoplastic (mast cell tumor in cats) ○ Septicemia/ Peritonitis/ Pyometra ○ Heartworm disease (cats) ○ Cholecystitis (cats) ○ Acute-on-chronic pancreatitis ○ Drugs – *same as left*
Dx	• 1st Tier: ○ PCV/TS ○ Blood smear ○ Blood Glucose ○ Azostix® (BUN) ○ NOVA/ I-Stat ○ Fecal float and sediment (zinc sulfate) ○ Fecal direct smear • Response to symptomatic care/ gastric rest: ○ Gastric Rest: · Withhold food & water for 12–24 hours. · Gradually reintroduce water. · Gradually reintroduce a bland diet. · Gradually transition back to normal diet after 3 days.	• 1st Tier – *same as left* • 2nd Tier: ○ CBC, Chemistry, Urine Analysis ○ ACTH-stim test (or baseline cortisol) ○ Abdominal radiographs ○ SNAP cPL or fPL® ○ SNAP Parvo® • 3rd Tier: ○ Abdominal ultrasound ○ Abdominal radiographs with contrast ○ Gastroduodenoscopy ± mucosal biopsy ○ Exploratory laparotomy ± PT/PTT (if hematemesis is present)	• 1st Tier – *same as left* • 2nd Tier – *same as left, plus:* ± Fecal float (zinc sulfate, q24h × 3d) ± Total T4 (cat >7 years of age) ± Heartworm Ag and Ab testing (cat) ± Gastrointestinal panel • 3rd Tier – *same as left*

- • Source: 8, 11

209

Sources Cited:

1. *BSAVA Manual of Canine and Feline Emergency and Critical Care*, Third Edition. Edited by Lesley G. King and Amanda Boag. © 2018 John Wiley & Sons, Inc.

2. *IRIS Staging of CKD*. © 2017 International Renal Interest Society (IRIS) Ltd.

3. *Plumb's Veterinary Drug Handbook*, Ninth Edition. Edited by Donald C. Plumb. © 2018 PharmaVet, Inc.

4. Prittie, J. (2006). Optimal endpoints of resuscitation and early goal-directed therapy. *Journal of Veterinary Emergency and Critical Care, 16*(4), 329-339. doi:10.1111/j.1476-4431.2006.00160.x

5. *Shock Pathophysiology*. Edited by Elizabeth Thomovsky and Paula A. Johnson. © 2013 Vetstreet, Inc.

6. *Small Animal Clinical Diagnosis by Laboratory Methods*, Fifth Edition. Edited by Michael D. Willard and Harold Tvedten. © 2012 Saunders.

7. *Small Animal Toxicology*, Second Edition. Edited by Michael E. Peterson and Patricia A. Talcott. © 2006 Elsevier, Inc.

8. *Textbook of Small Animal Emergency*, First Edition. Edited by Kenneth J. Drobatz, Kate Hopper, Elizabeth Rozanski, and Deborah C. Silverstein. © 2019 John Wiley & Sons, Inc.

9. *Textbook of Veterinary Internal Medicine*, Eighth Edition. Edited by Stephen J. Ettinger, Edward C. Feldman, and Etienne Cote. © 2017 Elsevier, Inc.

10. *The ABCDs of Small Animal Cardiology – A Practical Manual*, First Edition. Authored by Sonya G. Gordon and Amara H. Estrada. © 2013 LifeLearn, Inc.

11. *Emergency Procedures for the Small Animal Veterinarian*, Third Edition. Authored by Signe J. Plunkett. © 2013 Saunders, Ltd.

12. Goldberg, Katherine J. "Goals of Care: Development and Use of the Serious Veterinary Illness Conversation Guide." *Veterinary Clinics of North America: Small Animal Practice*, vol. 49, no. 3, May 2019, pp. 399–415.

Sources of Borrowed Images:

•   Pingstone, Adrian. Cycas Sago Palm. 2004. Wikipedia: The Free Encyclopedia. Wikimedia Foundation, Inc. Web. Accessed 5 January 2017. <https://commons.wikimedia.org/wiki/File:Cycas_Sago.palm.arp.750pix.jpg> (Public Domain)

•   Σ64. *Amanita virosa*. 2014. *Wikimedia Commons*. The Wikimedia Foundation, Inc. Accessed 8 January 2017. Web. <https://commons.wikimedia.org/wiki/File:Amanita_virosa_12.jpg> (CC BY 3.0)

•   Krisp, H. *Death Cap, Amanita phalloides*. 2013. *Wikimedia Commons*. The Wikimedia Foundation, Inc. Accessed 8 January 2017. Web. <https://commons.wikimedia.org/wiki/File:Grüner_Knollenblätterpilz_Amanita_phalloides.jpg> (CC BY 3.0)

"Because you are alive, everything is possible."
- *Thich Nhat Hanh*

CBC:

- **RBC** (10^6/µl): *D-RI*: 5.5-8.5; *C-RI*: 5-10
- **PCV** (%): *D-RI*: 37-56; *C-RI*: 24-45
  - *Mild Anemia:* D30 –37; C20–26
  - *Moderate Anemia:* D20–29; C14–19
  - *Severe Anemia:* D13–19; C10–13
  - *Very Severe Anemia:* D<13; C<10
  - *Anemia of Chronic Disease:* D25–35; C20–25 (normocytic, normochromic)
- **HGB** (g/dl): *D-RI*: 10-20; *C-RI*: 8-15
- **MCV** (fL): *D-RI*: 60-77; *C-RI*: 39-55
- **MCHC** (g/dl): *D-RI*: 32-36; *C-RI*: 31-35
- **RETIC** (/µl): *D-Regen*: ≥60,000; *C-Regen*: ≥50,000 aggregate
- **WBC** (10^3/µl): *D-RI*: 6-17; *C-RI*: 5.5-19
  - *Leukemoid Reaction:* >50,000–100,000 /µl (without leukemia)
- **NEU** (10^3/µl): *D-RI*: 3-11.5; *C-RI*: 2.5-12.5
  - *Corticosteroid Response:* ~15,000–25,000 /µl (<40,000 /µl)
  - *Require Sepsis Monitoring:* <1,000–2,000 /µl
  - *Presumed Sepsis:* <500–1,000 /µl and febrile
  - *Suspend Chemotherapy with Myelosuppressive Agents:* <2,500 /µl
- **BAND** (/µl): *DC-RI*: 0-300
  - *Inflammatory Disease:* neutrophilia with a left shift >1,000 non-seg/µl
- **LYM** (10^3/µl): *D-RI*: 1-4.8; *C-RI*: 1.5-7
- **MONO** (/µl): *D-RI*: 150-1250; *C-RI*: 0-850
- **EOS** (/µl): *D-RI*: 100-1250; *C-RI*: 0-1500
- **BASO** (/µl): *DC-RI*: 0-150
- **PLT** (10^3/µl): *D-RI*: 200-500; *C-RI*: 300-800; *Greyhound Dogs*: ~150
  - *Risk of Spontaneous Thrombosis:* >1,000,000 /µl
  - *Risk of DIC:* >50,000 /µl and patient is spontaneously bleeding
  - *Risk of Spontaneous Bleed:* <30,000–50,000 /µl
  - *Top Differential is IMT:* <50,000 /µl
  - *Suspend Chemotherapy with Myelosuppressive Agents:* <50,000 /µl
  - *Normal Cavalier King Charles Spaniel & Norfolk Terrier:* <10,000 /µl
- **TS-Plasma** (g/dl): *DC-RI*: 6-8

Urinalysis:

- **USG** (GMS/1000): *Dog-RI*: ≥1.030; *Cat-RI*: ≥1.035
- **PH**: *DC-RI*: 6.0-7.0
- **Protein** (mg/dl): *D-RI*: 0-30 or trace with USG >1.012; *C-RI*: Neg
- **Glucose** (mg/dl): *DC-RI*: Neg
- **Ketones**: *DC-RI*: Neg
- **Bilirubin**: *D-RI*: Neg or trace with USG ≥1.030; *C-RI*: Neg
- **SSA** (protein): *D-RI*: 1+ with USG >1.012; *C-RI*: Neg
- **Acetest** (ketone): *DC-RI*: Neg
- **Ictotest** (bilirub): *D-RI*: Neg or trace with USG ≥1.030; *C-RI*: Neg
- **Casts** (/lpf): *DC-RI*: 0-2 hyaline or granular casts
- **WBC** (/hpf): *DC-RI*: <4
- **RBC** (/hpf): *DC-RI*: <5
- **Bacteria**: *DC-RI*: Neg in cysto sample
- **Cells** (/hpf): *DC-RI*: 0-2
- **Crystals**: *DC-RI*: None to Few

- **Urine Protein/Creatinine Ratio (U/PC):**
  - *Non-proteinuric:* D<0.2; C<0.2
  - *Borderline proteinuric:* D0.2-0.5; C0.2-0.4
  - *Proteinuric:* D>0.5; C<0.4

Venous Blood Gas:

- **pH**: *D-RI*: 7.32-7.40; *C-RI*: 7.28-7.41; (7.1<☠>7.6)
- **PCO2** (mm Hg) *D-RI*: 33-50; *C-RI*: 33-45
- **HCO3** (mEq/L): *D-RI*: 18-26; *C-RI*: 18-23

Arterial Blood Gas:

- **pH**: *D-RI*: 7.36-7.44; *C-RI*: 7.36-7.44; (7.1<☠>7.6)
- **PCO2** (mm Hg) *D-RI*: 36-44; *C-RI*: 28-32; (☠>70)
- **HCO3** (mEq/L): *D-RI*: 18-26; *C-RI*: 17-22
- **PO2** (mm Hg): *D-RI*: ≈100; *C-RI*: ≈100; (☠<60)

Serum Biochemistry:

- **Glucose** (mg/dl): *D-RI*: 60-135; *C-RI*: 65-131; (40<☠>1000)
  - *Coma or Seizures:* <40
  - *Hyperosmotic diabetes with CNS dysfunction:* >1,000
- **Lactic Acid** (mg/dl): *D-RI*: 9.9-46.8; *C-RI*: 5.4-15.3
  - *Lactic Acid (mmol/L):* DC-RI: 0.22-1.44; (☠>6.0)
  - *Associated with poor prognosis:* >6.0 mmol/L
- **Cholesterol** (mg/dl): *D-RI*: 120-247; *C-RI*: 56-161
- **SDMA** (µg/dl): *DC-RI*: 0-14
- **BUN** (mg/dl): *D-RI*: 5-29; *C-RI*: 19-33
- **Creatinine** (mg/dl): *D-RI*: 0.3-2; *C-RI*: 0.8-1.8
- **Na** (mmol/l): *D-RI*: 139-147; *C-RI*: 144-155; (120<☠>170)
  - *CNS signs:* <120 or >170 in dogs
- **K** (mmol/l): *D-RI*: 3.3-4.6; *C-RI*: 3.5-5.1; (2.5<☠>7.5)
  - *Muscle weakness:* <2.5
  - *Cardiac conduction disturbances:* >7.5
- **Cl** (mEq/l): *D-RI*: 107-116; *C-RI*: 113-123
- **Na:K Ratio:** *Addison's suspect at* <27:1
- **Total Ca** (mg/dl): *D-RI*: 9.3-11.8; *C-RI*: 8.4-11.8; (7.0<☠>16)
  - *Tetany:* <7.0
  - *Acute renal failure and cardiac toxicity:* >16
- **Ionized Ca** (mmol/L): *DC-RI*: 1.12-1.42
- **P** (mg/dl): *D-RI*: 2.9-6.2; *C-RI*: 3.8-7.5; (☠ <1.5)
  - *Hemolysis, CNS signs:* <1.5
- **Ca×P Product** (mg/dL): *Mineralization at* >60
- **Mg** (mg/dl): *D-RI*: 1.7-2.1; *C-RI*: 1.7-2.3 (1<☠>10)
- **HCO3** (mmol/l): *D-RI*: 21-28; *C-RI*: 19-26 (☠ <12)
  - *Suspect severe metabolic acidosis:* <12
- **AG** (mmol/l): *D-RI*: 10-18; *C-RI*: 12-19
- **OSM** (mOsm/kg): *D-RI*: 290-310; *C-RI*: 308-335
- **TP** (g/dl): *D-RI*: 5.7-7.8; *C-RI*: 6.1-7.7
- **Albumin** (g/dl): *D-RI*: 2.4-3.6; *C-RI*: 2.5-3.3; (☠ ≤1.5)
  - *Severe hypoalbuminemia; at risk for major fluid shifts:* ≤1.5
- **Globulin** (g/dl): *D-RI*: 1.7-3.8; *C-RI*: 2.3-3.8
  - *Severe hyperglobulinemia:* ≥5
- **Bilirubin** (mg/dl): *D-RI*: 0-0.8; *C-RI*: 0-0.6
  - *Icteric plasma:* ≥1.5
  - *Icteric mucous membranes:* ≥3
- **ALT** (U/L): *D-RI*: 10-130; *C-RI*: 26-84
- **ALP** (U/L): *D-RI*: 24-147; *C-RI*: 20-109
- **GGT** (U/L): *D-RI*: 0-25; *C-RI*: 0-12

Other Diagnostics:

- **Systolic Blood Pressure** (mm Hg):
  - *Hypotensive:* <80
  - *Normotensive:* 90–140
  - *Prehypertensive:* 140–159
  - *Hypertensive:* 160–179
  - *Severely Hypertensive:* ≥180
- **Mean Arterial Blood Pressure** (mm Hg): *DC-RI*: 60–100
- **Central Venous Pressure** (mm Hg): *DC-RI*: 3–8

- **SpO2** (Pulse Oximetry – hemoglobin saturation with oxygen) (%):
  - *Normal:* ≥95

- **ETCO2** (Capnography – an estimate of PaCO2) (mm Hg):
  - *Normal:* 35–45
  - *Maintenance for traumatic brain injury patients:* 30–35

- **BMBT** (min): *Normal platelet function in D:* 2.6 ± 0.5
- **PT** (sec): Measures extrinsic and common pathways
- **aPTT or ACT** (sec): Measures intrinsic and common pathways
- **D-Dimer** (µg/mL):
  - *<0.25 has a strong NPV to (more or less) rule out DIC*
  - *>0.5 is characteristic for PTE in dogs (Se 100%; Sp 70%)*

- **T4** (µg/dl): *D-RI*: 0.8-3.5; *C-RI*: 1-4
- **Cortisol** (µg/dl): *D-RI*: 1-6; *C-RI*: 1-5
  - *Addison's suspect:* <2 (must perform ACTH-stimulation test)

- Key: *D* – dog; *C* – cat; *RI* – reference interval; *Regen* – regenerative; *Neg* – negative; ☠ – danger values
- Helpful Equations:
  - **RETIC (/µl)** = (RETIC[%]) × (RBC [10^6/µl])
  - **Corrected WBC count** = (NRBC × 100) / (NRBC + 100) [calculate if if nRBCs are >5]
  - **Corrected Total Serum Calcium** = tCa (mg/dl) – Albumin (g/dl) + 3.5 [Calculate if ↓ albumin; only in dogs >24 weeks.]
  - **AG** = [Na + K] – [Cl + HCO3]
  - **OSM (Osmolality)** = 1.86(Na + K) + (BUN/2.8) + (Glucose/18) + 9
  - **Osmol Gap** = measured OSM – calculated OSM [>25 mOsm/kg = presence of unmeasured osmols]
- Sources: 2, 6, 8; most CBC and serum biochemistry reference interval data are provided by the in-house Small Animal Clinical Pathology lab at the Texas A&M University Veterinary Medical Teaching Hospital

Emergency Drug Doses

Drug	Canine Dose	Feline Dose
Acepromazine	0.01–0.2 mg/kg, IV/ IM/ SC (maximum 3 mg)	0.01–0.2 mg/kg, IV/ IM/ SC (maximum 1 mg)
Apomorphine	1.5–6 mg, in conjunctival sac (for emesis) 0.03 mg/kg, IV; 0.04 mg/kg, IM; 0.02 mg/kg, SC (for emesis)	–
Atipamezole	3750 µg/m² BSA, IM (to reverse α2-agonists) 0.1 mg/kg, IV (to reverse α2-agonist in CPR)	Same
Atropine sulfate	0.04 mg/kg, IV/ IM/ IO (for CPR or atropine response test) 0.15–0.2 mg/kg, diluted 1:10 in saline or water, Intratrach	Same
Buprenorphine	0.005–0.03 mg/kg, IV/ IM/ SC, q6–12h 0.12 mg/kg, Oral Transmucosal	0.01–0.03 mg/kg, IV/ IM, q6–8h 0.03 mg/kg, Oral Transmucosal, q6–8h
Butorphanol	0.1–0.5 mg/kg, IV/ IM/ SC, q1–4h	0.1–0.5 mg/kg, IV/ IM/ SC, q1–4h
Butorphanol +Dexmedetomidine ± Ketamine	Butorphanol 0.4 mg/kg + Dexmedetomidine 0.005–0.01 mg/kg, mixed in same syringe and given IM (if no evidence of cardiovascular disease)	Butorphanol 0.3 mg/kg + Dexmedetomidine 0.005–0.01 mg/kg ± Ketamine 3 mg/kg, mixed in same syringe and given IM (duration of sedation is longer when ketamine is added)
Butorphanol +Midazolam +Other	Butorphanol 0.2 mg/kg, IV + Midazolam 0.2 mg/kg, IV + Alfaxalone 2 mg/kg, IV over 1 minute (provides excellent induction and recovery with minimal cardiopulmonary effects)	Butorphanol 0.4 mg/kg + Midazolam 0.4 mg/kg + Ketamine 3 mg/kg, mixed in same syringe and given IM (provides good sedation for physiologically-compromised cats)
Calcium gluconate (10%)	1 mL/kg of 10% solution (which corresponds to 100 mg/kg of calcium gluconate), IV slowly over 10–20 min (for treatment of hyperkalemia with K⁺ >8 mEq/L)	Same
Dexamethasone	0.07–0.14 mg/kg/day (anti-inflammatory), IV/ IM/ SC	Same
Dexmedetomidine	0.001–0.005 mg/kg, IV (or 125–375 µg/m² BSA, IV) 0.001–0.02 mg/kg, IM (or 165–500 µg/m² BSA, IM)	Same
Dextrose (50%)	0.5–1 mL/kg (0.25–0.5 g/kg), diluted 1:2 in sterile saline or water, IV slowly over 5 min (for treatment of hypoglycemia)	Same
Diazepam	0.5–2 mg/kg, IV/ Rectal/ Intranasal (for status epilepticus)	Same
Diphenhydramine	0.5–2 mg/kg, IV/ IM, q8–12h 2–4 mg/kg, PO, q8–12h	Same
Epinephrine	0.01 mg/kg, IV/ IO, q3–5min in early CPR (low dose) 0.1 mg/kg, IV/ IO, q3–5min in prolonged CPR (high dose) * 1:1000=1 mg/mL; 1:10,000=0.1 mg/mL	Same
Flumazenil	0.01 mg/kg, IV/ IO, q1h as needed (to reverse benzo's)	Same
Furosemide	1–4 mg/kg, IV/ IM/ SC, q1–2h	2–4 mg/kg, IV/ IM/ SC, q1–2h
Hydromorphone	0.05–0.2 mg/kg, IV/ IM/ SC, q2–4h (for analgesia)	0.05–0.1 mg/kg, IV/ IM/ SC, q2–6h
HES 6%	10–20 mL/kg, IV, given over 15–30 min (shock bolus)	5–10 mL/kg, IV, given over 15–30 min (shock bolus)
Hypertonic saline (7–7.5% NaCl)	4–5 mL/kg, IV, given over 5–10 min	3–4 mL/kg, IV, given over 5–10 min
Lidocaine†	2 mg/kg, IV, given over 2 min (for ventricular arrhythmia)	0.25–0.5 mg/kg, IV, given over 5 min (for vent. arrhythmia)
Mannitol	0.5–1 g/kg, IV, given over 10–20 min, q6h	Same
Methadone	0.1–1 mg/kg, IV/ IM/ SC, q4–8h (for analgesia)	0.05–0.5 mg/kg, IV/ IM/ SC, q4–6h (for analgesia)
Midazolam	0.1–0.3 mg/kg, IV/ IM/ Intranasal (for status epilepticus)	Same
Morphine	0.5–1 mg/kg, IV/ IM/ SC, given over 2 min, q2h (for analgesia)	0.05–0.4 mg/kg, IM/ SC, q3h (for analgesia)
Naloxone	0.01–0.04 mg/kg, IV/ IM/ SC/ IO (to reverse opioid)	Same
Packed RBCs	10 mL/kg, IV (1 mL/kg to raise PCV 1%)	Same
Plasma	6–20 mL/kg, IV, PRN for coagulopathy	Same
Prednisolone	0.5–1 mg/kg/day (anti-inflammatory), IV/ PO	Same
Procainamide	2 mg/kg, IV, given over 3–5 min, up to a total dose of 20 mg/kg (for atrial or ventricular arrhythmia)	–
Propofol	2–6 mg/kg, IV slowly to effect	Same
Terbutaline	–	0.01 mg/kg, IV/ IM/ SC, q4h (for asthma)
Whole blood	10–20 mL/kg, IV (2 mL/kg to raise PCV 1%)	Same
Xylazine	–	0.4–1.1 mg/kg, IV/ IM/ SC (for emesis)

† *Clinically-significant ventricular tachycardia*: ≥4 ventricular premature complexes consecutively at a rate of ≥160 bpm in dogs (≥240 bpm in cats)
• Sources: 3, 8, 11

Made in the USA
Monee, IL
08 April 2021